Wellness—
A Way of Life

By the same author

Martin, M.M. (2001) *Sustaining Health: The Physical Dimension in Health and Healing.* Saritaksu, Bali.

Martin, M.M. (1992) *Health and Healing from the Kitchen.* Pope Print, Timaru, NZ

Wellness— A Way of Life

Dr. Melva Martin

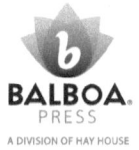

BALBOA.
PRESS
A DIVISION OF HAY HOUSE

THE HOLY BIBLE, NEW INTERNATIONAL VERSION®, NIV® Copyright © 1973, 1978, 1984, 2011 by Biblica, Inc.® Used by permission. All rights reserved worldwide.

Balboa Press books may be ordered through booksellers or by contacting:

Balboa Press
A Division of Hay House
1663 Liberty Drive
Bloomington, IN 47403
www.balboapress.com.au
1 (877) 407-4847

Because of the dynamic nature of the Internet, any web addresses or links contained in this book may have changed since publication and may no longer be valid. The views expressed in this work are solely those of the author and do not necessarily reflect the views of the publisher, and the publisher hereby disclaims any responsibility for them.

The author of this book does not dispense medical advice or prescribe the use of any technique as a form of treatment for physical, emotional, or medical problems without the advice of a physician, either directly or indirectly. The intent of the author is only to offer information of a general nature to help you in your quest for emotional and spiritual well-being. In the event you use any of the information in this book for yourself, which is your constitutional right, the author and the publisher assume no responsibility for your actions.

Print information available on the last page.

ISBN: 978-1-5043-1508-1 (sc)
ISBN: 978-1-5043-1512-8 (e)

Balboa Press rev. date: 10/23/2018

Dedication

Dedicated to all those individuals who seek knowledge and wisdom in order to discover that wellness is in fact a way of life. Also, to the people who read and made use of my earlier books and who still tell me how useful and valuable knowledge about those natural remedies has been in their lives. Finally dedicated to you, the reader, who may be seeking a reason for living a more abundant life, discarding the word 'sickness', and replacing it with 'wellness'

Contents

Foreword

"When the student is ready the teacher appears"

This is your moment. Here you are, holding a guide to better health and natural healing, written by an experienced naturopath who instructs the reader on inexpensive, home remedies that puts healing within reach of everyone. Well-rounded and thoughtfully compiled this guide addresses the triune: the body, mind and spirit. It is filled with effective approaches, doable techniques and treatments. Dr Melva Martin provides multiple options and paths to self-care. You may not choose to use all techniques included in this book, but you will learn the overarching aspects of health and holistic healing and find various treatment options to guide your journey forward.

If you are like me, you tired long ago of traditional, western, allopathic medicine that uses drugs to "treat symptoms" and was sometimes delivered with a bad bedside manner and the clock ticking. Worse yet, those drugs came with a list of alarming side effects and were often a temporary solution. My journey fueled by ill health as a child caused me to seek out alternative health care at an early age and what was within the realm of what I could do for myself. My doctors were not healing me and I was no dummy, so I got to work and it has truly paid off over time. You might be thinking, "I am not smart enough" but trust me this is not as hard as you might imagine. Melva boils it down into absorbable pieces for her readers.

The days of us leaning back and expecting a doctor with fifteen minutes to fix us is over. Worse yet, good health seems harder to achieve in our chemicalized world. Therefore, it is time for us to step up and get in relationship with our bodies and learn what we can do for ourselves before we resort to a medicine or surgery for every malady along life's highway. The reality is that no doctor will give us unlimited time and when we go to them we are wise to partner with them rather than passively sitting on the sidelines. Who else cares deeply about our health and that of our loved ones? We have the capacity to track, learn and grow as the baseline provider of our health. We live in our skins and can sense what works and what doesn't. The more proactive and involved we are improves our ability to work in concert with our doctors and practitioners. We no longer expect them to have all the answers and do all the work because we are taking responsibility for our own health and we are tracking along the way. I won't deny that there is a place for allopathic, western medicine, but it is time to return most of the care to our homes, our prayers, our kitchens and our gardens. This book will be your reference and your guide.

Melva teaches the basics of holistic health. The great triune of the body, mind and spirit. She begins with our connection to the macrocosm or our place in the energetic and spiritual realms. This is what I call the "quantum physical soup". She does not offend by speaking from only one religious tradition but speaks to spiritual and energetic connections as means for better health. She emphasizes the importance of ingesting pure water, reminding us that our bodies, like the planet are predominantly comprised of this essential component. She includes methods of using water in its various forms: liquid, ice and steam as external applications such as baths and packs.

Dr Martin's book offers a variety of time tested traditions. One chapter explains the use of the practice of homeopathy, how "likes" in micro dilutions treat "opposites", i.e., super dilated caffeine would treat insomnia. The best part is that homeopathy is perfect for children, the elderly, those with allergies or even a pet. Handy chart formats are included for easy reference. Another safe tactic included in this book are the Bach Flower Remedies, made from just that, flowers. They are a pleasant and subtle way to treat self and others, especially children and for emotional maladies. I especially like and use the Rescue Remedy that is readily available in health shops and pharmacies everywhere. Essential oil use is included. The most popular form of massage, Swedish, is described in substantial detail. Touch, the first sense to develop in utero, is always welcome and has benefits beyond the obvious physical ones. Skin to skin contact can produce the essential ingredient of healing: hope, comfort, caring and strength in a world of cold handshakes and pats on the back. Homeopathy, Bach Flower Remedies, aromatherapy and massage are powerful; approaches that require little or no effort on the part of the recipient and it often empowers the "patient's" willingness to try other remedies and begin an arduous healing journey.

If all these subjects aren't enough Melva is an avid gardener and self-sufficiency expert. She will work the tail off anyone half her age. She is spry and "walks her talk" as they say in the Native American tradition. Sustainability is norm. She farms her worms, composts all her food and yard waste, always has a new planting project underway and she maintains her excellent health by growing most of her own food. No grass grows under Melva's feet! This book will teach you techniques to improve the nutritional value of your garden crops and shows you how to grow food in a small space. This book also includes information on growing, collecting and using herbs and food as a part of a healing protocol.

Having spent forty years researching and applying alternative and holistic health techniques in an effort to improve my own health and fifteen years as a founder and CEO of one of the largest professional schools of massage in Dallas, Texas; I find this book to be a well-rounded manual for caring for your body temple while living this short time on Planet Earth. This book is chock full of skills and knowledge and perhaps a few reminders of healing concepts once read and then forgotten. I know that I did. Our life is a journey and health is only one of the aspects, but if we don't have good health, it can squash our dreams. Your focus may shift between prevention or natural treatments, you will find both within *Wellness a Way of Life.*

When we wake up and realize that no doctor can make us well without us doing our part is the day that wellness rises on the horizon. We cannot control the World but we can take control of significant aspects of our health by learning a few techniques, starting our gardens, practicing our skills and taking personal responsibility for our health.

All the best to you, the reader, on your journey to a richer, happier, healthier life.

Muriah Williams
Founder and CEO of *Wellness Skills*, Dallas & Fort Worth, Texas, 1985-2000. Vice Chair of the *Advisory Council, Texas Health Department, Massage Therapy Division* 1987-1993.

Preface

My journey through life has taken me along many, many paths - some good, some not so good, some sad, some joyful. However, I believe that through every experience in life there is a reason, or a higher purpose that is being fulfilled. I trust that this book will provide help for your journey to wellness, and that it may demonstrate that you do not always need to take drugs and medicines to sustain health.

Once upon a time when I was a small child we lived in the country and never saw a doctor. Coughs, colds, influenza, mumps, chickenpox, measles came and went as part of life. There were no antibiotics and our mother were both our doctor and nurse. Generally, if we were sick, we were sent to bed and administered copious lemon drinks, salt gargles for sore throats, and onion and honey syrup for coughs. Broths, malt, molasses, and herbs were our tonics to get us well fast. We soon got better and were outside running barefoot in the fresh air and sunshine.

Growing up on a farm there was no time to be sick because everyone had jobs to do, even children were kept busy helping their parents. We lived off the land – we grew all our own vegetables, strawberries, blackcurrants, gooseberries, and picked lots of blackberries in season from the roadside. Although our orchard was small, we had generous neighbours who shared their seasonal fruit with us. Everyone helped pick large amounts of fruit - most of which was then cooked and preserved to eat throughout the year. Fields of potatoes were grown which served our dinner table for a full year. Our father butchered animals, and our cows supplied us with fresh milk and cream. We made our own butter. Pigs fed with curds and whey (from cow's milk) grew to become pork and bacon. Eels and small crayfish were caught in the creek and on many occasions a rabbit was trapped. Hens and ducks supplied us with eggs and some were roasted, with herbed stuffing, and graced our table on special occasions.

Back then country people helped each other out. Neighbours shared the work of haymaking, which enabled everyone to get their hay stacked quickly in dry weather. Horse driven mowers cut the hay and helpers turned and stacked it with pitchforks. For morning and afternoon refreshments, women provided freshly baked scones with billies of tea.

Social events were held in a local hall and musical evenings were held in different homes of those who were musically inclined. If anyone left the community, there was always a farewell gathering with music, dancing, a fabulous supper, and in conclusion, farewell speeches and gifts. Children joined in and learned to dance too.

Children ran around barefoot, skillfully climbed trees, swam in creeks, ran up and down hills, watched birds, cared for orphan lambs, raised calves, grew their own vegetable gardens, rode horses (and cows), rode bicycles down dusty unsealed roads, and lived a relatively carefree existence close to nature – strong and well.

Memories of childhood are part of who I am. I have always had a yearning to be back with my bare feet on the land and now, having completed a whole cycle of living, I'm back on land growing my own food and aiming to become self-sufficient once again. To me this is an important pathway to wellness and a way of life that I am guided to share with you, a seeker of better health.

However, I know that it is not possible for everyone to live on the land and to be totally self-sufficient. It has taken me many years to get to where I am now, but I have followed a path, even in the city, that has been a way of wellness – that is, living without resorting to drugs or spending lots of money on expensive 'natural health' supplements. Growing nourishing vegetables and herbs is an extremely rewarding experience – anyone, anywhere can do it!

Do you want *a way of life without pharmaceutical drugs and other prescription medicines*? A way of life where you can be in control? A way of life where you can determine the steps that your future journey takes you? A way of life without fear, without stress, and without side effects from pharmaceuticals? A way of life filled with energy, excitement, joy, challenges, and unexplainable reward? How do I know? I have lived more than 40 years without ever having touched a drug for either pain or sickness. I have quality of life and try to live what I impart, and I know these *basics* are the essential starting points for anyone seeking a new start in life and living well. My greatest desire is to integrate almost fifty years of experience and knowledge into a useful format so that the reader, and all whom they care for, will have a life of robust health and happiness.

This book is written for those who seek another way to live either with pharmaceutical drugs within the 'medical' or 'disease' model in relation to health, or, alternatively within a 'wellness model' whereby prevention and reversal of disease is possible without drugs. Reversing signs and symptoms of disease *is possible* when viewed through a wellness model. Let's think and talk wellness! and be well…

Acknowledgements:

I am eternally grateful to God the great Spirit 'S' who created the universe and all its beauty and to all the beautiful people in this world whom I have met on my journey through life.

From the beginning of life people mold our character. Some people and events will leave a mark in our memory forever. There are times we cannot understand the 'why' but later in life it becomes clear. To all things there is a purpose and a reason as there is a season. I am grateful for the people who taught me the knowledge and skills of various kinds and with those I have experienced, (and still do) the wonderful adventure of life. Many members of my family and friends have passed on as have teachers and acquaintances… to you all I am deeply grateful.

Special thanks to Margaret and Cindy for reading various drafts and contributing suggestions for this book. To my nephew Calvin and colleague Muriah who proof read and provided valuable comments for the final draft. Thanks to Franzi who managed to create a beautiful *Wellness Model* from my sketches.

Introduction

We travel through life like a ship on the sea. Every ship will be blown about by the wind and tossed by the waves, yet a stable and strong ship can sail with the winds and find direction through obstacles confident that it will reach its destination safely. We can set our course and stick to it, or we can be diverted to whatever and wherever any whim may take us. We can collapse when challenges come our way or embrace them and find a way through. We choose how we travel through life and how we are guided. We can be positive, successful, and satisfied along our course, or we can become negative, do the wrong thing and end up in a mess. Everyone makes mistakes and it is through our mistakes that we learn, gain experience, and are able to help one another along the way during our journey through life.

Natural Health implies that the human body has the capacity to sustain health and to heal itself. Natural Health Therapies prevent most forms of sickness and have the ability to treat and heal alongside mainstream medicine. Of course, a misplaced broken bone cannot be fixed by natural therapies alone for it is best set in place for the bone to heal properly. At the same time an herbal (comfrey) or homeopathic remedy (symphytum) can be taken to accelerate the healing process in a natural way.

As far as natural health thinking goes, all healing is self-healing according to natural laws. Numerous studies have demonstrated the ability of the mind to control the body and the environment is seen to affect emotions. Loving, caring relationships enhance wellness. Religious and spiritual beliefs maintain a connection with that deep spiritual core or essence that is timeless within the human body and has the power to heal mind, emotions, and the physical body

Within these pages you will discover many pathways to sustain wellness and a range of effective treatments for you and your loved ones if you are sick. These methods and remedies have stood the test of time and no effort will be made here to argue their efficacy or present the results of empirical research proving this efficacy. This is a way of life that many have chosen, it is not expensive, and can lead to wellness and good health.

Chapter One introduces a holistic approach to health, healing, and the history of natural cures. The concept of wellness gained through nature cure laws is introduced.

Chapter Two explores the spiritual core or essence of the individual as the immortal part of the mortal body and ways of connecting to the Divine and the related healing powers of belief.

Chapter Three explores ideas about spirituality and models of health and wellness.

Chapter Four provides information about water, its importance for sustaining health, and usefulness in sickness.

Chapter Five is about fasting and the importance of minerals in the body.

Chapter Six introduces food and diet and explores approaches to eating and ways to manage food allergies and sensitivities.

Chapter Seven is an introduction to energy medicine and describes the system of homeopathy. Several homeopathic remedies are suggested as first aid for sickness or injury.

Chapter Eight describes the discovery of the Bach Flower remedies, their preparation and application to emotional problems.

Chapter Nine covers herbal remedies and their usefulness at home. Several are described that are readily available and how they can be used in everyday life to keep you well or as a resource for treating ailments.

Chapter Ten is an introduction to Aromatherapy (essential oils), and how they can be used to strengthen and harmonize the body.

Chapter Eleven begins an introduction into the value of touch as a healing modality and presents a practical way to use massage techniques to relax and balance the body.

Chapter Twelve is about foot therapy and covers metamorphosis and zone therapy with methods of using foot reflexes to effectively produce change in another part of the body.

Chapter Thirteen is devoted to starting a journey towards wellness by sustaining health through growing your own nutritious vegetables and herbs.

Chapter Fourteen discusses one of the most powerful practices of healing and maintaining wellness by connecting with the great Spirit of the universe (God). Also, vibrational sound and how to use the voice for healing and maintaining wellness.

Chapter Fifteen suggests self-help routines and exercises to incorporate into daily activities, as a way of life, on the journey to wellness.

CHAPTER ONE

Wellness – A Way of Life

Wellness is a WAY of LIFE - it is a lifetime experience. Here you will discover the basics that you need to know to start your journey into wellness. As you help yourself you will be able to help your family, neighbours, friends, and the many people who cross your path. Nothing here is new a lot is common knowledge passed down from generation to generation and you will find advice that a traditional naturopath would provide. Complementary and alternative medicines and methods will provide a range of choices from which you can select the most appropriate to use in your wellness journey throughout life.

Don't worry if you slip up every now and again, we all do! We are imperfect mortal human beings and, although we strive for the best, sometimes we do fall short. BUT get up and get going again, and again, and again, NEVER GIVE UP!

If you are really sick then you may need to initially consult a medical doctor, naturopath, or natural medicines practitioner.

The history of the Western medical profession is recorded to have originated in antiquity as part of Greek and Roman cults associated with various deities that healed the sick. Apollo was recognized as the god of healing but, strangely enough, in some cults, he was also considered to be the god of ill-health and plagues. Hippocrates of Kos (circa 460 to circa 370 BC) is generally considered to be the first healing practitioner to believe that diseases were not the result of superstition and vengeful gods, but caused naturally by a combination of environmental factors, diet and

1

habits. He separated the discipline of medicine from religion and turned to diet and herbs for healing.

Hippocrates came to be known as the 'Father of Modern Medicine' and he wrote about *'vis medicatrix naturae'* – the healing power of nature, and *'natura medica'* – natural cures. This was the beginning of a tradition of nature cure therapists who, since that time, have endeavoured to work with healing forces present in nature and within the human body. Traditional naturopaths have always maintained a holistic philosophy and treat *people* rather than symptoms and diseases. Traditional naturopathy has evolved over time and today contemporary naturopaths are also called natural medicines practitioners who diagnose and prescribe natural remedies in a similar manner to a medical doctor who diagnoses an illness and prescribes pharmaceutical drugs.

A natural medicine practitioner will make a diagnosis and prescribe from a wide range of herbs, natural medicines, and nutritional supplements to treat the problem. Remedies may be costly to the client. Natural medicine and supplementation is an industry which has become big business akin to the pharmaceutical industry, and most pharmaceutical companies now produce 'natural' supplements too! A naturopath or herbalist generally no longer makes up herbal medicines such as capsules and potions for the individual in the traditional manner. Today a prescription can be taken to a health food shop or pharmacy where the remedy is purchased.

As with pharmaceutical drugs natural medicines can have side effects, especially high potency supplements. Also, there is a risk involved taking some natural medicines with pharmaceutical drugs. A discussion should always take place with either your pharmacist or medical doctor if you intend taking both pharmacy medicine and natural medicine together.

There are still practicing *traditional* naturopaths around who prefer to work without prescribing medicines or high potency supplements and they will generally start by looking closely at an individual's diet and nutrition. Hippocrates was a firm believer in good nutrition and one of his popular sayings is still quoted today: *"Let food be thy medicine and medicine be thy food"*. People are becoming more aware that what they eat affects their health, especially with the relationship of a high sugar intake to an increased incidence of diabetes and obesity in Western and Pacific Island countries.

Current research demonstrates that a high sugar intake is related to an increased incidence of diabetes, obesity, and cardiovascular diseases. As people start to think more for themselves and realise that self-healing is a reality and self-help care is possible then people often become more discerning in their choices related to food. The future will be one of survival drawing on the traditions of the past by those who take control of their health - seeking to live a long and active life exempt from disease.

The medical profession has always focused on diagnosis and treatment of diseases yet today a wholistic approach to health and wellness is becoming more common. The approach of practitioners may be with drugs or other technical methods. Alternatively, the diseased part of the body is surgically removed. There are, of course, major advantages of surgery and many lives have been saved through the skill of surgeons, for example, the benefits gained from surgeons who repair broken and traumatised bodies after car accidents. Also, in cases where the vital force of the individual is unable to reverse the process, for example a ruptured, inflamed and infected appendix - removal of the appendix and infected tissue is life-saving in most cases. We can never discount the work of the medical and surgical professions, as these are good people who have a calling and do a tremendous amount of excellent work. It is misuse of expensive pharmaceutical drugs that cripple the economy of a country and often compromise the health of people including over prescribed or self-administered pharmaceuticals, or side effects from them.

Today, power over the health sector lies with pharmaceutical drug companies, the medical profession, and political interests. People rely upon their doctor and prescription drugs to treat their ailments and make them well. Unfortunately, one drug often leads to another, and another, as a person's condition progressively deteriorates, and in the end, a person may be even more unwell than before as drug side effects surface. Most drugs have effects and side effects and often a patient will die from the side effects of a drug or a combination of drugs rather than the disease!

Being alerted to side effects of a drug will enable a patient to determine whether they are experiencing side effects from the drug or if their disease is getting worse. You are the expert of your own body and the way it functions. In a fifteen-minute consultation it is impossible to convey all information about yourself to a doctor. It is time to become educated about pharmaceutical drugs and know their effects and side effects. It helps to always read literature that comes with every prescription. Some side-effects are cause for immediate attention. Don't be afraid to ask questions or discuss your concerns with your doctor either about your illness, the drugs prescribed, or possible side-effects.

The medical and drug bill for New Zealand escalates as more and more people suffer lifestyle and chronic diseases and are treated within the medical model with drugs. Patients who have been treated with antibiotics for years no longer respond to them so there is a growing concern about how to treat these sick people who have developed antibiotic resistance.

Medical doctors who try turning people away from taking prescribed drugs and follow more natural ways are often ostracized by their peers, or not considered good doctors by their clients. Many people are addicted to this way of life and have faith that doctors and drugs are the answer to all their problems and they may become upset if their doctor does not prescribe them something. Yet many patients have experienced much better health, and even reversed disease - such as cardiovascular disorders, obesity, and diabetes - by turning away from pharmaceutical drugs and towards more natural medicines and therapies such as nutritional advice, and regular physical activity.

It is often only courageous and strong-minded people who can break themselves free from drugs and the medical model and try something different. Forward thinking doctors and nurses working within a wholistic model for health may encourage their clients to take 'green prescriptions' rather than (or as well as) pharmaceutical prescriptions whereby clients can take advantage of health promoting community programs using local facilities. The green prescription may include guest speakers talking about wellness, swimming in a community pool, dancing to music (in or out of a swimming pool), and various gymnasium exercises to suit the individual. These activities are provided free or at a reduced cost to the client in their community environment. Activities may be carried out in groups where each client's vital signs are monitored by a nurse, before and after exercise, to ensure there is a gentle slow progression back to an improved state of health, without harm.

However, there *is* another way. There *is* hope and there *is* a path to wellness and happiness without pharmaceutical drugs with a reduction in drug dosages over time. It is possible with the right attitude and the right program to reverse disease.

Naturopathy as we know from a traditional viewpoint, is a means of maintaining health and treating disease by following the principles and laws of 'nature cures'. The traditional naturopath seeks to assist the patient in restoring the vital energy within their body. One way the body's natural healing ability can be enhanced by another person is by using their hands doing reflexology, zone therapy, or metamorphic techniques on the feet or by doing body massage. Any treatment with a helper using their hands is considered healing touch therapy. Self-help methods such as massage and zone therapy are techniques that are easy to learn and will be discussed in later chapters.

Traditional remedies and methods are simple, well tested, and are very effective. They have stood the test of time and are cost effective. The philosophy and beliefs of traditional naturopathy are simple and follow principles of 'nature cures' whereby laws of nature follow patterns as described below.

Eight basic natural laws are:

> The concept of *vital energy;*
> The *self-healing body;*
> The *rule of the artery is supreme*;
> The *accumulation of waste in the body* causes disease;
> *Healing takes place from the centre to the outside of the body*;
> The *last symptom to appear will be the first to disappear* as healing takes place;
> A *healing crisis* will occur before total healing takes place;
> A person in *harmony (mind/body/emotions/spirit)* is healthy and well.

Now let's take a look at each of these ideas and explain them a little further.

Vital energy

Vital energy is the life force that flows through the body. This has always been acknowledged within natural therapies and is needed for the optimal function of the body. Other terms used when discussing this 'vital energy' energy are 'Chi', 'Prana', and 'Chakra energy'. There is a great deal written in books about energy flows from Chinese and other traditional healing practices. Blockages or imbalances of natural energy can manifest as signs and symptoms of disease, which may be specific to a particular tissue or organ of the body, or a deficiency may simply manifest itself simply as lack of energy. Disease can nearly always be reversed if the vital energy of the body has not fallen too low!

The self-healing body

The human body has all the essential elements within it to repair and heal. If the body is supported naturally, its self-healing powers will enable it to recover quickly from fatigue and sickness and maintain both balance and wellness. Symptoms of pain or disease may disappear almost miraculously by administering painkilling drugs, but the body is not healed. The person is free of symptoms, yet the disease has not had the chance to heal naturally or completely. Pain is a warning sign indicating a problem needs attention. Drugs will eliminate pain but the disease may be suppressed.

Generally, a suppressed disease shows up later as either the same pain, or as an illness on the same or a deeper level within the body. In other words, a skin rash due to stress may be treated with a corticosteroid cream for years and the rash will disappear when the cream is applied yet it will always return. Much later irritable bowel syndrome may surface that is related to the original stress causing the skin rash (and not diagnosed as stress related) showing that a completely different problem has arisen.

If the body's self-healing power is restricted by ignoring stress responses or due to poor nutrition the chances are that the person will eventually suffer symptoms of pain or disease. As a person becomes more aware and conscious about why he/she is not well, he/she will often come to realise, from within, the correct action to take to become well. Supporting the self-healing energy within the body will facilitate wellness.

The rule of the artery is supreme

The rule of the artery is supreme means that a good clean blood flow through the arteries is important to nourish all cells and tissues of the body. The cardiovascular system carries blood, through arteries, to every cell in the body in order to nourish the cells. Blood needs to be of a certain consistency with adequate nutrients and water to prevent blood becoming too thick or too thin. If blood becomes thick and sluggish it may clot and cause problems and if the blood becomes too thin a small cut may be hard to stop bleeding.

Blood also needs to keep moving along arteries and veins and that requires physical activity, movement and exercise.

The accumulation of waste products in the body causes disease

Disease occurs when the body is overloaded with toxic or cellular waste products which may be the result of poor dietary decisions, smoking, environmental pollution, or pharmaceuticals stored in the cells and tissues of the body. For example, when the body cannot keep up with processing and metabolising food adequately, end products stored in the bowel result in constipation - faeces are not eliminated and the body tends to reabsorb some fluid waste back into the body. Smoking cigarettes, living or working in a polluted environment without fresh air, will result in the lungs becoming coated with toxic material that eventually causes disease. When illness is suppressed with pharmaceuticals and the cleansing organs such as the liver and kidneys are not functioning well, stored waste products eventually reach joints, muscles, and brain cells.

When the body is not given the proper care it needs to deal with waste products, the final sickness is generally the last one in a whole trail of illnesses. Breathing fresh air helps the lungs eliminate toxic material. Exercise and drinking adequate water assists the body to deal with toxic waste material. A well-functioning digestive system with a daily bowel movement regularly rids the body of waste.

Healing takes place from the center to the outside of the body

With nature cure methods the human body is considered as a whole (other terms are wholistic or holistic). Toxins naturally begin to be stored in the skin where they cannot do too much harm away from the vital organs i.e. the heart, liver, and lungs. As more and more toxic material builds up in the body, joints and organs become affected. When healing occurs, the vital organs at the center of the body such as the heart, liver, and lungs will be given priority over the skin so they are always healed first. Often a skin condition will remain for years because it will be the last to heal. This is what is meant by healing from the center to the outside of the body.

The last symptom to appear will be the first to disappear with healing

Healing is a process. Healing is cyclic and there are often many ups and downs before a full healing occurs and the person is well. The general rule with healing is that the last symptom to appear will be the first to disappear. Illness can build upon illness unless something is done to intervene and set the body on a recovery pathway to wellness. To enable the body to heal itself, the body will first remove the illness that occurred last, subsequent to the previous illness, and so forth until all illness has been overcome and the body is healed and well again. At each stage during the process there will be ups and downs as the body heals itself so one must be patient and not give up.

A healing crisis will occur before total healing takes place

The human body is constantly trying to maintain a state of harmony and balance. We use the term homeostasis to define a static state of balance within the body and the term homeodynamic to define a more dynamic on-going state of wellness. A healing crisis occurs during this homeodynamic healing process. During the healing crisis an individual's vital energy assists to remove waste products from his/her cells and tissues. A higher than normal state of energy is often the first sign that a healing crisis is about to begin.

Sometimes the cleansing organs cannot keep up with the overload of waste products present in the bloodstream. Therefore, waste products will remain in the organs and tissues until the cleansing organs have caught up. This waste toxic material may have been stored for months or years. When a healing crisis occurs toxins are released into the bloodstream to be excreted from the body through organs such as the lungs (sputum), kidneys (urine), skin (sweat), and bowel (faeces).

Knowing the difference between sickness and a *healing crisis* is important.

When a healing crisis begins often a person thinks he/she is ill but in fact this is not always correct. A healing crisis commonly starts as a headache with symptoms similar to a cold or influenza. *Before* a healing crisis an individual will have plenty of energy because the vital force is at work gathering energy before the healing crisis begins. Also, during a healing crisis the person may experience their most recent illnesses or symptoms. Although these signs and symptoms may be similar to sickness, the body is really doing great work healing itself. That is why it is important to understand the healing process, so the individual can assist their body to heal with natural cures.

During a healing crisis it is time to rest, to drink plenty of fluid, or to fast on fruit, vegetable juices, or broths, to breathe fresh air, to exercise in moderation, and to think positive thoughts in order to encourage the body to recover in every way possible. If at all concerned during this time, consult your health practitioner or someone who understands the working of the human body, the effect of nature cures, and the healing crisis, in order to help you understand what to do. Often it is good to be monitored during this time for support and reassurance.

Fasting to detoxify or eating very little food may facilitate a healing crisis. Eating only one type of food such as grapes or watermelon will encourage the body to detoxify and eliminate toxic material through the liver, digestive system and kidneys. Taking a bath with a cupful of Epsom salts will help eliminate toxins through the skin.

A person in harmony is healthy and well

If a person functions with their body, mind, emotions, and spirit, all in a balanced state and in harmony within their environment, they should be healthy and well.

CHAPTER TWO

"Seek and you shall find the kingdom of God within you"

Jesus (Luke Ch. 17v21)

The following chapter describes the foundations of my personal spiritual journey mainly based on the Christian faith and my study of universal religions. I appreciate that many readers of this book may have discovered and explored life's spiritual dimension through a completely different journey that may draw on completely different faiths and religious traditions. I acknowledge that every individual's spiritual journey is equally legitimate as mine.

In the beginning...

"God created the heavens and earth".[1] God made man and woman to care for the earth, the birds, the animals, every creeping thing, and all that is upon the earth. Science and religion provide us with some answers but, for many people, how we believe the world began, and how we found our place in it, and our purpose on earth is mostly beyond comprehension. We live by faith and the knowledge scientists are now discovering.

In the *Holy Bible,* and elsewhere,[2] where Spirit is referring to God, Yahweh, or Jehovah, the word Spirit begins with a capital letter "S" and where spirit denotes the human spirit, the word spirit begins with a small case letter "s".

"We know that we live in him and he in us because he has given us of his Spirit."[3]

In the *Acts of the Apostles*, Paul provides this explanation for God ('S') to describe humanities role in relationship to the living God 'S'.

"The God who made the world and everything in it is the Lord of heaven and earth and does not live in temples built by hands. And he is not served by human hands, as if he needed anything, because he himself gives all men life and breath and everything else. From one man he made every nation of people that they should inhabit the whole earth and he determined the times set for them and the exact places where they should live. God did this so that men would seek him and perhaps reach out for him and find him, though he is not far from each one of us. For in him we live and move and have our being."[4]

I think Paul was striving to explain that this was a living God 'S' and humankind 's' was a part of this divine universal energy in which we "live and move and have our being". Wayne Teasdale, in his book *The Mystic Heart*[5], concludes from studies of universal religions and natural mysticism that everything is within God. In his book he uses the term "Panentheism" (not to be confused with "pantheism") whereby he explains that everything is within God, in the consciousness of the divine or the divine mind. Many mystics, religious devotees, and others have grasped this idea yet many, particularly in Western cultures, view God or the Divine as something external to themselves.

Does the spiritual part reside at the core of our being or somewhere else? My faith, reflection, and experience in life leads me to believe that yes, indeed, the spiritual part lies within the core of our physical body and yet is an essence that permeates our whole being. Our spirit is capable of connecting throughout our total environment to energise our physical body and sustain wellness. During research conducted while monitoring cranial rhythms of volunteer spiritual healers and healees, the author discovered that during the process both healer and healee had significantly reduced cranial rhythms. I speculated that in some way this cranial rhythmic impulse is associated with the spirit 's', which is linked to, and reflected from 'S'. I believe the spiritual part of our humanness ('s') connects with the greater universal energy or God ('S'). This idea ties into Luke's statement where he quotes Jesus as saying: "The kingdom of God is within you."[5]

Humanities predominant belief is that spirituality, as a concept, can be interpreted in different ways from various 'holy' scriptures, fields of research, and individual experience. For example, Teasdale[6] brings eastern ideas of spirituality into a western Christian perspective and he suggests that God, the divine reality of Christianity, is the source of all that is and connects all beings, all reality, and life together. Similarly, Nakagawa[7] from the Buddhist tradition, informs us that the ultimate reality that is Buddhism is similar to Christianity and he sees an interconnectedness of all sentient beings through all religious beliefs. Nakagawa brings western concepts into eastern ideas to form his multidimensional theory and he suggests that it appears to be this interconnectedness and self-connectedness with spiritual elements that is important for health and wholeness. Spirituality is present within a range of religious belief systems as well as outside religions as in the act of healing the self through a relationship with the divine.

Considerable discussion in education has been about spiritual intelligence and the measuring of what has been termed a Spiritual Quotient (SQ) which is in line with the more familiar Intelligence Quotient (IQ) and Emotional Quotient (EQ). SQ (Spiritual Intelligence) is new concept and probably unknown to many even though there is enough collective evidence from psychology, neurology, anthropology and cognitive science to show that there is a third intelligence, an SQ which is unique to humans and is associated with love.[8]

Love is a word that is interpreted and expressed in many ways. The *Oxford Dictionary* defines love as "deep, intense affection; sexual passion; a beloved person or thing."[9] The *Holy Bible* says "God is love"[10] In *Science and Health with Key to the Scriptures* we read: "Love, the divine Principle, is the Father and Mother of the universe, including man."[11] Jung wrote: "Man can try to name love, showering upon it all the names at his command, and still he will involve himself in endless self-deceptions. If he possesses a grain of wisdom, he will lay down his arms and name the unknown by the more unknown… by the name of God."[12]

The ancient Greeks believed that love was the domain of Eros, a god whose divinity transcended human limits and could not be represented in any particular way and love was not always fuzzy and nice. In our modern age Owen[13] points out that love itself has hard edges, particularly in moments of transformation and he views love as having two faces – a face of acceptance and a face of challenge. Through total acceptance, love is experienced by accepting people for exactly who they are. However, *love of acceptance* is balanced by *love as challenge* whereby the very best is expected – being the best that one can possibly be. This does not mean conforming or achieving to someone else's marker but rather about a personal best and wholeness.

Love has nothing to do with judging another, or informing another that they don't love themselves enough, or that all their problems are related to an unloved childhood. Love is an expression that can be freely given and accepted in many different ways.

Unconditional love is the ability to love without ceasing and without judgement. It is the *Golden Rule* in action – 'Love God with all your heart, mind, body and spirit and love your neighbor as yourself.' Total love casts out fear and heals. Words spoken with love have a powerful effect on humans, animals, plants and will be discussed in a later section on water (Emoto's[14] research). Larry Dossey in his book, *Healing Words - The Power of Prayer and the Practice of Medicine.*[15] points out that love is intimately related to health and that the power of love is legendary, built into folklore, common sense, and everyday experience. Love connected with prayer or thought can reach out to heal at a distance – akin to telepathic law. Over and over again it has been demonstrated that love, compassion, and caring facilitate healing and it is perhaps the greatest power that can regenerate and revitalize. As Dossey says, "Love occupies a majestic place in healing. Lying outside space and time, it is a living tissue of reality, a bond that unites us all."

The heart is often viewed as the centre of love where the divine spirit dwells. The experience of 'heartbreak' (from whatever cause) can be felt as physical pain in the chest where the heart is situated. Upledger[16] indicates that the pericardium constricts when emotional issues are not resolved, and he demonstrates that this can be treated in a natural manner through energy release techniques and unconditional love. Dawson Church[17] has added ideas from experimental research about the relationship of heart, mind, and matter to unconditional love. He proposes that emotional freedom techniques (EFT), can tap into matter and energy meridians, in order to release mental and emotional problems that restrict the individual from developing their full potential. Dawson Church and others, from a scientific background, demonstrate an approach in which an individual can not only change themselves through their related consciousness of the universe but also change their environment.

From my own experience after the sudden death of my son I experienced severe chest pain. I thought I was about to have a heart attack. Relief came through prayer, love of friends and family, and a puppy that came into my life with unconditional love.

Love permeates all: it is an energy, it is infinite, it is linked to the spiritual side of life (God is love).

"…if there is a natural body, there is also a spiritual body… For the perishable must clothe itself with the imperishable and the mortal with immortality."[18]

In accordance with Paul's explanation, the spirit 's' is at the core of, or emanating from, the physical (mortal body) and is more significant than the physical part of an individual… it is ME…it is the "I AM"… it is forever ME. It is powerful and eternal. In Western Christian mysticism there is a sense of an indwelling spirit linked to the source of all things, a point at the center of a human that belongs to God, 'S', which is indestructible and eternal. "Don't you know that you yourselves are God's temple and that God's Spirit lives in you?... for God's temple is sacred and you are that temple."[19] St Paul has much to say about love including the following: "Love is patient, love is kind. It does not envy, it does not boast, it is not proud. It is not rude, it is not self-seeking, it is not easily angered, it keeps no record of wrongs. Love does not delight in evil but rejoices with the truth. It always protects, always trusts, always hopes, always perseveres. Love never fails."[20]

All this being true, as the apostle Paul says the physical body still needs to be taken care of if it is to be considered a sacred temple in which the spirit resides.

Religious beliefs attempt to explain spirituality but often doctrines of a church can confuse one on the journey to spiritual fulfilment. A church is simply a community of people of the same faith or belief system (and often the same cultural understanding). Many people find their questions answered, as well as spiritual comfort and fellowship within a church community. For some people, the exclusivity of a specific church group is a deterrent to spiritual growth. Serious Christians will hold what is actually written in the *Holy Bible* above any religious principles or doctrines promulgated by a given church or denomination and will seek to demonstrate the life of a disciple as a follower of Jesus. Many people follow a spiritual path without the need to belong to a church or similar group and this is a personal choice.

A Christian is basically a follower of an Essene Jew called Jesus of Nazareth. Jesus was a humble man of prayer who saw all people as children of God, Yahweh, Jehovah, 'S', without exclusion and whose actions showed a way of love, peace, health, grace, mercy, and wholeness. He is reported to have performed miracles, cast out demons, and healed people, showing a way of service that his disciples could follow. Whatever he did, he said we could do it too, and his mission was to show a way of salvation and spiritual growth through service and peaceful living. Without discrimination, he valued the role of women, and saw the poor and outcasts of society as people worthy of acceptance and healing. Finally, through his death and resurrection he demonstrated new life and eternity.

"The Spirit himself testifies with our spirit that we are God's children"[21]

How do we know whether we have that closeness of the Spirit connected to us? Probably two words sum it up - love and peace - which is demonstrated through "fruit of the Spirit - love, joy, peace, patience, kindness, goodness, faithfulness, gentleness, and self-control."[22]

Humans are like a tree – feet connected to Mother Earth, arms raised to Heavenly Father and heart in harmony with other humans. The symbolic *Tree of Life* found in many cultures reflects this idea. When an individual experiences closeness to Spirit peace resides within the human spirit and fruits of the Spirit become evident. Often others experience that on-flow of love and peace that comes from God through the eyes, words, and deeds of those living close to Spirit. Lives that demonstrate love and peace, are expressing their spiritual nature. Gabriel Cousens writes about "peace by being peace"[23] a wonderful philosophy and something to strive for in the chaotic world around us. Every individual can make a difference in their environment by connecting to God 'S', being kind, loving, and expressing attributes of the spirit 's' that contribute towards peace.

Many religious and spiritual groups have as core values love of God (the creator) and love of neighbor (which is everyone). Expressions of love are loving thoughts, words, and deeds, and a joyfulness that gives meaning to life and living. If everyone practiced these values the world would be at peace; everyone would have sufficient for their needs, everyone should be happy and able to communicate in harmony, accepting and appreciating one another's differences. In Paul's letter to the *Galatians* he says: "... serve one another in love". The entire law is summed up in a single command: "Love your neighbour as yourself".[10]

Since we live in an imperfect world, life is often a struggle, particularly with a low inflow or outflow of love. To overcome our imperfections each one of us can contribute by doing our bit within our immediate environment. Being well is composed of a positive approach, attitude, outlook, and delight in daily living. Conversely, negativity, sickness and sadness destroy and take away life. Because we are imperfect we will make mistakes. However, we learn from our mistakes and often become able to lovingly help others along their path to wellness because of what we have learned from our own mistakes and challenges, and how we survived and overcame them. We hopefully learn to forgive, through acceptance of diverse viewpoints and loving kindness, when others hurt us or treat us unkindly. Within our environment we have opportunities to improve ourselves and our relationships with others, trusting that this will have a ripple effect from families, to circles of friends, and into the community to each and everyone we meet, and on into the world. What we do makes a significant difference.

Love is an energy. A person with loving thoughts creates an energy field that affects other people, animals, and anything within their immediate environment. Consider loving thoughts and prayers reaching long distances. Absorption of love energy heals. A person may not be aware that they are producing healing energy with their physical or non-physical presence (as in a phone call, a conversation, or intentional loving thoughts) yet the recipient of the energy will be affected in some way. Intentional healing imbued with loving thoughts, is more powerful than most realise.

It is indeed a tremendous blessing to be a disciple of a spiritual teacher, yet not all have discovered such a person and are still seeking. However, it is also possible to grow spiritually from reading and contemplating the writings of spiritual persons, philosophers, or those making direct contact with God's Spirit and putting into practice lessons learnt. Praying,

17

meditating, and listening to the still small voice of the spirit within our very being – sometimes called intuition helps us along the way too.

What exactly is *spirituality*? It can be defined as the an active, personal, and experiential process that connects one human spirit one with another that also links with God's Spirit. Human's connect in dialogue and the *voice* of two persons can be consider a spiritual experience. (Voice and sound will be discussed in a later chapter). Danah Zohar and Ian Marshall[24] write about a spiritual quotient SQ. Just as intelligence is measured by an IQ, and emotions measured by EQ, spirituality is measured by SQ. Their belief is that SQ originates in the deep center of the self, grounded in all the infinite potentiality of energy that has no beginning and no end.

Jesus of Nazareth came into the world with a specific purpose (as we all do). His purpose was prophesised in the *Old Testament* of the Hebrew Scriptures (*Holy Bible*). Jesus came as the Messiah in order to show humans a way of love, peace, and power that leads to eternal life. after three years of preaching, teaching, and healing, it cost him his life on the cross. The *New Testament* informs that there are many other works that Jesus did which are not recorded.[25] Other writings, including those by Pliny the Younger, Josephus, and within the *Dead Sea Scrolls,* confirm *Holy Bible* stories about the life of Jesus and his works. Jesus declared that his purpose was to teach people about life, how to live it abundantly, and by his death and resurrection demonstrated that our spirit is eternal.

Jesus was a Jew, a wanderer, and a social reformer. He chose twelve to be apostles and help with his work. He drew many disciples to his way of life and living and walked amongst all kinds of people teaching about love, peace, and the kingdom of God. He is known to have grown up in an Essene community where he lived a simple life close to nature. The Essenes and the first Christians were teachers and healers who lived an orderly life abiding by laws of nature. They understood how to utilize earth, sun, water and air to grow food and keep healthy. They were vegetarians and sprouted seeds to eat and to make bread, they worshiped, prayed, and meditated morning, noon, and night. As followers banded together after his death they formed churches to support one another and they performed healings just as Jesus commanded:

"Go into all the world and preach the good news to all creation…

these signs will follow those who believe… they will place their hands on the sick people, and they will get well."[26]

The practice of healing as Jesus taught did carry on after his death and in the early churches, but today is largely lost except in those countries where faith in the power of God is strong and pharmaceutical drugs unobtainable (as in parts of Africa). In most western countries today, pharmaceutical drugs are first choice treatment for sickness rather than faith in the power of God to heal. However, many people who have been healed will testify that the Spirit of God ('S') still heals today.

Personally, I received laying on of hands with prayer after fracturing my spine (X-ray evidence of fracture) several years ago, I experienced a powerful instantaneous healing with disappearance of pain. I knew instantly that I was healed by this powerful Spiritual energy. Since then I have never experienced any trouble with my back. In my clinical practice I have seen many people healed in this manner. I have listened to many stories about healing through faith and prayer alone as well as laying on of hands for healing. In many cases *faith* alone heals the sick person - faith in God, faith in the practitioner, faith in the medicine or treatment. Faith where love is present is powerful – a loving husband or wife, parent, friend, professional, or simply a loving caring touch all have a huge impact in the healing process.

So, if the laying on of hands was common practice around the time of Jesus, then what happened? Throughout history political and church powers have tried to control people in many ways. Many healers, herbalists, and midwives were murdered, often being labelled as witches and sorcerers. All they were doing was making people well and keeping them healthy. Many followers of Jesus who proclaimed the gospel message and healed either hid or gathered secretly, while others declared their faith and died as a result.

Today prayer for healing or laying on of hands is generally free within some churches. Some practitioners who call themselves spiritual healers will charge for their service, yet many spiritual healers give freely of their time. Many medical and other practitioners heal as Jesus healed in their own quiet way without proclaiming that they are spiritual healers. With faith one can heal oneself and with faith another can heal. So why don't more people take advantage of this method of healing? Someone said to me once, "Perhaps it is because people lack knowledge and are not ready for a spiritual experience." Maybe that is correct, maybe people do not realise they can be healed through prayer or other spiritual experiences. Perhaps by sharing this knowledge prayer and hands on healing will become a way of life for many who embrace this wisdom. To experience ways of connecting with Spirit is firstly, to have an understanding and an awareness of our own spirit and how we relate to God (Spirit).

Prayer, contemplation, meditation, music and singing, are widely held ways to connect with God. In a group situation this can become a very powerful and energizing experience, particularly when praying, singing, or chanting. There are many other ways to connect with God including through free gifts the creator has provided. Let's take a look at some of the free gifts from God that enables us to connect with Spirit in order to experience peace and healing.

Sunrise and sunsets – colour/light.

Fresh air and oxygen - absolutely essential for life.

Birds – sound and beauty: music for the soul.

Flowers – beauty, colour and aroma.

Trees – beauty, colour, grounding.

Animals – unconditional love.

Butterflies, bees, and insects – beauty and colour.

Water and streams – essential for life, beauty, sound.

Weather – rain, frost, snow, sunshine, clouds, wind.

Earth – essential to grow grass, food, and barefoot grounding.

Stars - beauty, light, cosmic energy.

Moon - beauty, light, rhythmic energy.

Humans – fellow spiritual beings that bless us in many ways – a touch, a hug, a tone of voice, a word, a glance, a helping hand when in need.

We experience individual gifts of creation in many ways – listening to music, viewing art, doing work, or just sitting in the silence listening to God ('S').

There is a lovely old song that many children learn to sing at an early age which reflects the work and greatness of God in the world:

All things bright and beautiful,

All creatures great and small,

All things wise and wonderful,

The LORD GOD made them all.
Each little flower that opens,
Each little bird that sings,
He made their glowing colours, He made their tiny wings.
The rich man in his castle,
The poor man at his gate,
God made them, high or lowly, And ordered their estate.
The purple-headed mountain,
The river running by,
The sunset and the morning,
That brightens up the sky; -
The pleasant summer sun,
The ripe fruits in the garden, -
He made them every one;
The tall trees in the greenwood,
The meadows where we play,
The rushes by the water,
We gather every day; - He gave us eyes to see them,
And lips that we might tell
How great is GOD Almighty,
Who has made all things well." [27]

CHAPTER THREE

A Wellness Model

To be well is to be alive

Now that we have viewed sickness and wellness from a conventional and nature cure viewpoint and also explored some ideas about spirituality let's take a look at current health and wellness models that attempt to define health and provide guidelines for daily living.

The World Health Organisation (WHO) definition of health[28] is as follows:

*"**Health** is a state of complete physical, mental and social well-being and not merely the absence of disease or infirmity."*

Models of health in New Zealand include three Māori health models promoted by the *Ministry of Health*[29]:

Mason Durie developed two health models: *Te Pae Mahutonga* and *Te Whare Tapa Whā*. Let's now explain these models a little further:

Te Pae Mahutonga (based on the Southern Cross Star Constellation) brings together elements of modern health promotion with the four central stars of the Southern Cross representing key tasks of health promotion, i.e. Mauriora (cultural identity), Waiora (physical environment), Toiora (healthy lifestyles), Te Oranga (participation in society) with the two pointers of the Southern Cross representing Nga Manukura (community leadership) and Te Mana Whakahaere (autonomy).

Te Whare Tapa Whā brings together four cornerstones of Maori health: Taha tinana (physical health), Taha wairua (spiritual health), Taha whānau (family health) and Taha hinengaro (mental health). The view is that if foundations are strong and four sides equal then the person is healthy. If any one of the four dimensions is missing or damaged a person, or a collective, may become 'unbalanced' and subsequently unwell.

The third is a model developed by Rose Pere – *Te Wheke*. The **Te Wheke** model (the octopus) shows that traditional Māori health acknowledges the link between the mind, the spirit, the human connection with whānau, as well as the physical world in a way that is seamless and uncontrived. The idea of Te Wheke is to define family health. The head of the octopus represents Te whānau (the family), the eyes of the octopus Waiora (total wellbeing for the individual and family), and each of the eight tentacles represent a specific dimension of health that is interwoven: Wairuatanga (spirituality), Hinengaro (the mind), Taha tinana (physical wellbeing), Whanaungatanga (extended family), Mauri (life force in people and objects), Mana ake (unique identity of individuals and family), Hā a koro ma, a kui ma (breath of life from forbearers), Whatumanawa (the open and healthy expression of emotion).

A Wellness Model (Figure 1) was developed by a New Zealander with Celtic cultural roots. This perspective demonstrates a holistic way to view health and wellness. The *Wellness Model* begins with a circle (representing eternity in Celtic lore). The circle brings into the model natural dynamics representing the circular nature of life and living. It represents the great Spirit 'S' or source of all, permeating all things ("in which we live and move and have our being").

At the centre, and radiating outwards is a representation of the individual, the immortal spiritual ME, the I AM, the spirit 's' which is a spark of the greater Divine Spirit 'S'. Each spirit 's' is clothed with a human physical body. The diagram shows a channel reaching upward and outward and downwards but in fact the spiritual energy permeates throughout everything. This model demonstrates that we are a small part of something much greater. In a sense it is a universal consciousness to which we are all connected. Individually, our immortal spirit 's' is a spark or reflection of the greater 'S' the Divine, God, Spirit – light, love, or energy, that links to, or, reflects that which is greater than our individual self 's'. Everything is connected by the vibration of sound and colour.

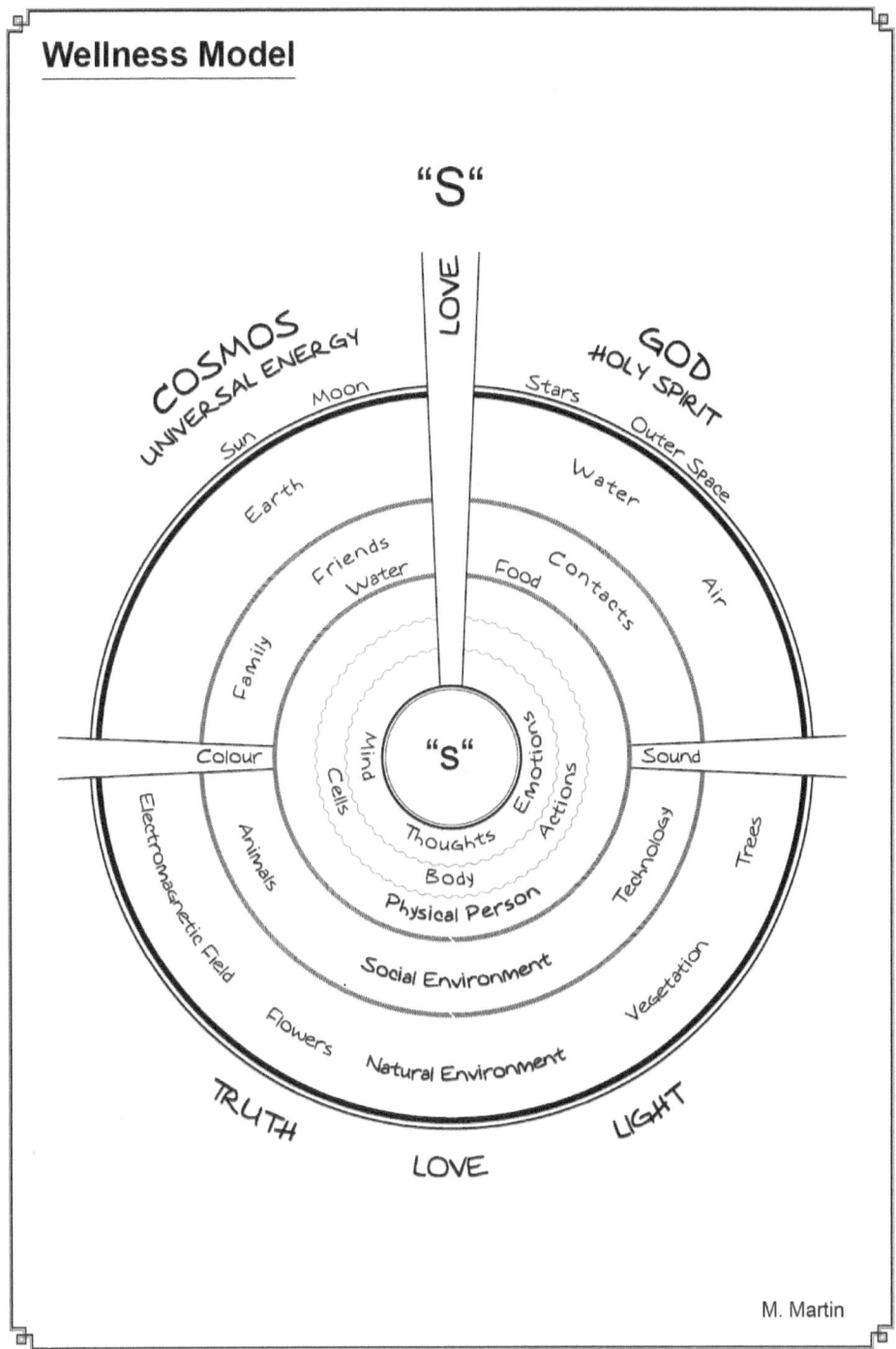

Figure 1: A Wellness Model

As we go beyond that which can be seen with the human eye we can experience an awareness of electro-magnetic and other universal energies from the earth, sun, moon, stars, and into infinity. These too can continue to be represented in never ending circles.

There are many, many, factors that relate to wellbeing, and the *Wellness Model* (Figure 1), although rudimentary, shows how we can view the individual 's' in a wholistic manner in relation to Spirit 'S' within our environment. When the universe's good, God energy, such as 'love' or 'light', permeates all it will influence wellbeing and harmony, health, and healing. With unconditional love all is possible.

An additional support to the understanding of this *Wellness Model* added here is a pattern of *Celtic Circles*. This diagram of five folded circles is associated with the balance of the universe.[30] The circle in the middle represents the universal Spirit 'S', while the four circles surrounding it represent the four elements: earth, sun(fire) water, and air. This symbolic representation illustrates how the four elements are intertwined and interrelated and in doing so keeps the universe in balance. It also represents the symbol of connectedness and unity between all things.

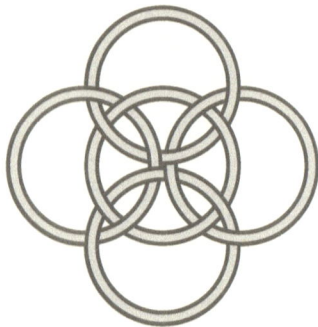

Figure 2: Celtic Circles: a Pattern of Connectedness and Unity

Spirituality

We might talk about our *experience* of Spirit in many different ways. Whatever we name it, we receive the breath of life from Spirit at birth that enables us to become a living human being. The spiritual aspect is expressed through a human mortal body and we experience life.

From the moment of conception, a human being becomes a bundle of cells that continue to divide and grow and form tissues and organs resulting in a physical body and born as a human being. It is as if the mortal body is the clothing that lasts until the time of death. At death the immortal spirit 's' sheds the mortal physical body and the immortal spirit or soul leaves. The mortal body returns to the basic mineral elements from which it was made and becomes dust. At death, the physical body has done its job. Just like clothes that wear out and get discarded the physical mortal body disintegrates and all that is left behind are pictures and memories in the human minds of those mortals who are still living on earth.

Meanwhile the 'I AM', ME, or 's', the spiritual soul moves on… into the realm of whatever faith and belief the person conceives the after-mortal life to be. Some people have been 'to the other side' and have come back to tell their stories. Those who have gone 'to the other side', are now reassured about the life to come. Others simply live by faith in the love of 'S' and the belief that they will be taken care of eternally and that there should be no fear of death when the mortal body dies as the spirit 's' continues to live 'on the other side'.

This all adds up to an immortal spirit 's' clothed with a physical body that radiates energy, electricity, light, colour, and sound. It has been written that the eye is the lamp of the body. The eye reflects the light and spirit of the immortal soul.[31]

The liturgy in the *New Zealand Prayer Book* is an inspiration for many people as they connect and communicate with God, other people and the environment… "we whom the Spirit lights give light to the world… we, filled with the Spirit's grace and power, may be renewed for the service of your kingdom" [32]

Energy from the universe is known to connect with an energy source in the human body called a 'chakra' system. This system transmits vibrational energy throughout the physical body and infuses every part of the body with energy. This energy can be related to the vibration of colour as well as musical notes. In a similar manner breathing allows the human body to absorb oxygen from universal air when inhaling (inspiration), which is then distributed throughout the body. After an exchange process, within the body, waste carbon dioxide is released back into the atmosphere when exhaling (expiration). All these processes occur according to nature's laws whereby humans benefit from energy systems in the environment.

Plants and trees benefit from carbon dioxide released into the atmosphere by humans and humans benefit from oxygen released by plants and trees. Therefore, getting close to plants and trees and talking to them and breathing with them can be of value to both humans and plants and sitting under trees or beside plants is very therapeutic. The vibration of colour from plants and flowers has a therapeutic effect on humans, and energy from sound (voice or music) has been shown from research to benefit plants too.

Many standard models of health care focus on the physical body which, of course, is easier to study than the mental, emotional or spiritual dimensions of a human-being. Today in the western world people are conditioned to seek medical advice for anything that affects the physical mortal body (including mind and emotions). It is difficult for most people to understand that there might be another, more effective, way to deal with sickness and health challenges. Often, as a last resort people turn to alternative therapies, or spiritual healers, and are pleasantly surprised to find they *can* get results from those who have sometimes been called 'Quacks'

Going back to the *Wellness Model* in Figure 1. We know that the environment influences everyone on earth. If a person lives in a positive loving environment, then there is more likelihood of that person being well rather than if they lived in a negative environment. Factors involved in social environments are relationships with other people - family, friends, work colleagues, contacts at social events etc. Imagine if everyone in the world believed in loving kindness and peace and set out to follow the *Golden Rule* to love God 'S' and love their neighbor 's' as themselves!

Domesticated and wild animals, birds, and insects all have an influence on the well-being of humans. Any other aspect within the natural environment will also affect well-being. Trees, vegetation, flowers, and the electromagnetic field of the earth also influence wellbeing. Some ways to reverse negativity or depression and to feel good are to love and stroke a pet, love and hug a tree, experience the colour and beauty of a pleasantly perfumed flower, or watch a bird or insect at work.

The influence of the earth, sun, moon, water, and air are all important for wellbeing. People get sick if the air is polluted with smoke or chemicals, they get depressed if they don't see the sun or become ill if they work in buildings without windows and are drinking toxic water.

Finally, the known and unknown cosmic relationship to the earth affects the wellbeing of humans. The Greeks used the word Kosmos to describe the whole of existence – not just matter (lifeless and unfeeling) but the living totality of matter, body, mind, soul and spirit.[33] Planet earth is a very small part of the cosmic environment and it emits cosmic radiation that affects human beings and their environment. Seckely[34] suggests that although we live in an era whereby radiations may be harmful to optimal vitality of humans we can be assisted with good radiations from the earth, sun, moon, water, air, those factors can be of immense value to health and healing. For example, knowledge of natural laws such as planting vegetables in parallel with cycles of the moon provides an optimal environment for plant growth and enables humans to harvest nutritious and energized food.

Technology generated radiations from television, cell phones, and other modern equipment may be harmful to humans and can affect wellbeing. Don't despair, there are ways to detoxify and prevent harmful radiations affecting the body. With Tachyon technology[35] it is possible to protect oneself from negative radiations and be well. One of the simplest and best ways to eliminate harmful radiation or balance the body after being exposed to too many positive ions is to walk barefoot on the earth and/or grass or walk upon sand along the seashore. This is an excellent 'grounding' technique and enables an individual to connect with the source of all and eliminate the detrimental effects of radiation from the body by allowing earth energies to deal with it. Another method to disperse harmful radiation from office or household technology is to have green and flowering living plants inside and to place spagnum moss in jars or vases close to objects such as television sets which are likely to emit harmful radiation.

Charles Fillmore[36] views creation as a trinity like process. He reflects and proposes that behind the visible universe the original creative force (Yahweh/Jehovah/God) and the cosmic rays crystallize into earthly things. By understanding this trinity and its various truths we should be able to reconcile discoveries of modern science with fundamentals of religion. The idea of electrical thought forms can be compared to the link between God 'S' and a person 's'. If the circuit is clear the energy will flow, all things will be possible. Fillmore applies this natural law to humankind (s), God (S), and prosperity, yet it can just as effortlessly be applied to health, wellness, and wellbeing. To explain a little further - life in the body is like electricity in a motor: life is the energy that propels the body into action and the force behind life is the 'vital energy'. The pure life of Spirit 'S' flows into mankind's consciousness through his/her spiritual body, 's'.

In a similar manner Celtic Christianity[37] views life in its totality. Everything is sacred, creation is good and blessed, and there is no such thing as 'secular' and 'religion' being separate streams of thought or action. Spirituality is wholistic and a way of life to live because all things remain in God 'S'.

Wellness as a way of life agrees with elements of traditional Celtic Christianity that takes into account our natural environment, and the way we live, work, connect, and function within this environment. By aligning our spiritual self 's' with the creator 'S', by utilizing the laws of nature and cosmic energies, and by applying ancient and current knowledge in a wise and beneficial manner wellness can be achieved. Love is the great connector and the bond that unites, heals, and sustains the pathway to wellness.

LOVE expressed and received is a key to wellness.

CHAPTER FOUR

Water The Best Medicine

Take your Medicine until you need no Medicine at all

People taking medicine, prescription or otherwise and who believe they cannot live well without it may be hesitant about making changes. Unfortunately, some prescription drugs become addictive and it is difficult (and sometimes unwise) to suddenly stop taking them. Pharmaceutical drugs such as prednisone, if taken for any length of time may cause nasty side effects and if suddenly discontinued may cause serious life-threatening problems. Anyone considering reducing or stopping prescribed medication should first *discuss with their health practitioner.* Nowadays, it is easy to use the internet to find out if a drug is addictive, has side effects, and whether it is safe to discontinue. Always make an informed decision and consider your choices carefully.

If you have made the decision to try something different and are on medication, be wise and reduce the medicines slowly if possible. Discuss your plan with your medical doctor or pharmacist who prescribed the medicine. Perhaps you can take a smaller dose or take every other day. Everyone is different and may have different starting points on the road to wellness when attempting to reduce medication.

There are many common complementary therapies that can be used alongside drugs or can be taken instead of some drugs. Know that some herbal remedies may interact with pharmaceutical drugs thus wisdom and good guidance is essential.

Water and its importance to life

We are born with about 90% water in our body, but the volume of water tends to reduce with age. Unfortunately, many disorders are the result of dehydration and are not recognized as being related to lack of water. To be well and in an optimal state of health, adults should maintain at least 70% water within their body fluids, so it is essential to drink adequate amounts of water daily.

The therapeutic effects of water are known, for example, a headache is a common symptom of dehydration or lack of water. Many illnesses can be cured with water alone as has been demonstrated by Dr Batmanghelidj's[38] research.

In his book *Your Body's Many Cries for Water*, Dr Batmanghelidj tells his remarkable story. Prior to 1979 he was involved in completing a family charity medical centre in Iran but, during the revolution that followed he was imprisoned and all personal and family assets were confiscated. The authorities were preparing to execute him. The revolutionary guards realised that he could perhaps be useful as a resident doctor among the prisoners, so his execution was delayed.

Late one night one of the prisoners experienced severe abdominal pain and was diagnosed with a peptic ulcer. Dr Batmenghelidj was called to treat him. There were no medicines available so in desperation he prescribed two glasses of water. It worked – within eight minutes the pain disappeared. According to Dr Batmanghelidj it was at this point in time a new era in the advancement of medical science was born as he realised the value of water. During the next two years while in prison he researched the medicinal value of water, particularly for the use of reducing stress related diseases among the prisoners.

The day of his trial came, and Dr Batmanghelidj was required to answer to 32 fictitious indictments carrying the death penalty. As a final defense he presented the judge with an article on water treatment for peptic ulcer disease. Remarkably, his life was spared so that he could continue his research. The article (written in prison) was eventually published in the *Iranian Medical Council Journal* in 1982. In June 1982 he was released from prison and escaped from Iran to live in America. In 1983, the *Foundation for the Simple in Medicine* was formed in America to foster research into the topic of water to heal diseases.

In 1992 Dr Batmanghelidji was invited back to Iran where he addressed professionals at Tehran University and in teaching hospitals. He was also allowed to broadcast his views on television. Today the Iranian public is continuing to test the simplicity with which water can cure many medical problems. For example, he demonstrated that high blood pressure (hypertension) can be the result of an adaptive process to a gross body water deficiency and responds well to an increased water intake.

Dr Masaru Emoto, a Japanese scientist, is another well-known water researcher. During his studies Dr Emoto photographed frozen water crystals[39]. He experimented with many kinds of water and discovered the purer the water, the more beautiful the crystals.

Emoto then took his research further. He talked to water, played music to water, prayed to dirty water in order to clear the water, he wrote words on water jugs and stuck pictures on bottles of water. From all this research he discovered water had an amazing ability to react to words, music, pictures and even thoughts. For example, he wrote or said "Thank you" to one bottle of water and "You fool" to another bottle of water. The crystals showed a difference with the most beautiful crystals being the ones nice words were spoken to. If we relate to this research we can understand why the way we speak to one another and the music people listen to, can be uplifting or not. Water in the body can enhance wellness by the way we deliver and react to words, tone of voice, and sounds.

Emoto discovered that beautiful crystals came from water that flowed from mountain springs and streams – rainwater that naturally filtered through rocks and the earth. He concluded that because we are at least 70% water and because of this fact the *essence* of a human being is water. By taking into our body good clean water, speaking nicely to one another, and listening to uplifting music; we can expect to improve and sustain health and wellness.

Water constitutes all body tissues, yet it must be kept moving to be effectively used in the body. Water without movement can lead to functional problems in the body. Exercise circulates body fluids delivering nutrients to cells and removing cellular waste.

Drinking Water
Drinking clean water is important at all times but particularly in times of fever and dehydration. This is true particularly in hot climates, when

engaged in sports activities, or swimming in water for any great length of time. Constipation may result from drinking insufficient water. Extra water needs to be taken when suffering with diarrhea because this is a situation when the body quickly dehydrates.

During normal days drink sufficient water but do not force yourself to drink more than you personally feel comfortable about drinking. People have been known to force themselves to drink water and consequently drink much more than their body can tolerate. Tissues become water logged and the delicate natural chemical balance in their body is upset with the result that they can become unbalanced and disoriented!

Contrary to some beliefs about hot drinks made with water, such as tea and coffee, they still hold value as water. Water is still reaching body cells – cups of tea still count as water! However, as with any kind of drink whether it be tea or coffee with a caffeine content, high sugar fizzy drinks, or alcoholic drinks, excess can be harmful.

To know if you have been drinking enough water, take a look at your urine. Normal urine should be a pale straw colour. The less water you drink the more concentrated and stronger the colour will become (dark yellow or orange). If you are taking drugs or supplements observing your urine is not a good guide because chemicals from drugs and supplements may change the colour of your urine.

Some people are concerned about chemicals added to public water supplies to destroy pathogenic bacteria. As our drinking water gets more and more polluted we need to find a way to provide clean water and that means doing something about it ourselves. Water treated with chemicals such as chlorine kill bacteria. The outcome of this is the release of trihalomethane, a poison. Add to the water lead or copper from pipes through which water flows and there is more toxic material in the water by the time it reaches a drinking tap. Chlorine can be dispelled by boiling the water before drinking but fluoridated water is a different matter. Fluoride is added to water to prevent dental caries in children yet excess can cause a white mottled effect on teeth. Some adults are extremely sensitive to fluoride and this causes health problems. Chemicals and drugs are not removed from tap water unless people use a filter to do so.

It is highly recommended to have some kind of water filter to eliminate all pollutants such as fluoride, lead and copper (from pipes), trihalomethane (from dead bacteria), and anything else polluting the drinking water supply. One of the best ways to filter water is to utilise charcoal or an active carbon filter.

Eating organic fresh fruit and vegetables will always provide a source of natural water with nutrients. Consider how much water comes from watermelon, grapes, pineapples, and oranges. This is natural water with the addition of vitamins and minerals too!

Hydrotherapy

Water therapy or hydrotherapy has been used as a natural treatment since the beginning of time. Water is both soothing and stimulating on the body and is useful for practically all kinds of conditions. Best of all it is compatible with the human body because of the body's water content.

For centuries humans all over the earth have known about the therapeutic effects of bathing. Many hot mineral pools and spas are found in different countries. Natural springs have been known to be associated with spiritual and physical renewal, and there are places called 'holy' springs where healing occurs.

In New Zealand some precious waters come from the mountains, through many miles of underground aquifers, and pop up as fresh, cool, healing water springs. Also, hot mineral springs from the earth are found in Rotorua, Taupo, New Plymouth, Morere (East Coast), and in the Far North, as well as Hanmer Springs and other places in the South Island. Many are used for bathing and therapy.

Incidently, one of the Bach Remedies called Rock Water is not a flower, but is water from a natural spring. Rock Water, found in areas untouched by civilisation is said to be exposed only to sun and wind as it bubbles up among trees and grasses. It is known for its power to heal the sick and is one of the 38 *Bach Flower Remedies (see chapter eight)*.

Water used in hydrotherapy may be in one of water's three states: as a solid (ice), a liquid (water), or as a vapour (steam). As a liquid it can be cold, warm, or hot. Each form of water and its temperature range can be used specifically in various ways, internally or externally, either daily or as needed to sustain wellness or in a therapeutic manner to promote healing.

Historically, British and European Nature Cure Therapists treated many conditions with water only, both internally (fasting, douches, enemas) and externally (spas, sitz baths, aix massage, hot and cold packs, body wraps etc.). Care must be taken with both very hot water and ice as they both burn the skin if used incorrectly.

Hydrotherapy is a delightful way to enable your body to function well, both inside and outside, and a marvelous way to start the day refreshed and empowered.

A quick start to the day - drink a glass of pure water then walk outside on dew-covered grass.

The Cold Water Dash (hot and cold water)

As an alternative to your daily warm shower you may wish to start every day with your normal warm shower finishing off with a dash of cold water. Slowly adjust to cold water by introducing it slowly, a little every day. Some people enjoy a cold shower and some people have no option but to shower and bathe in cold water. In most OECD countries[40] a warm/hot shower is normal. If a hot shower is the usual routine, then switching to cold water can initially be a bit of a shock to the body.

Always begin with a warm body. This means, always ensure that you have warmed up sufficiently before adding cold water and do not stay in cold water too long. Try the cold-water treatment after your routine shower. You may need a bit of courage for the first few days. Once you have conquered the first few days, you may never want to finish your shower again without cold water! However, don't linger.

It is surprising how quickly hypothermia can take over the body while in cold water. Signs of hypothermia are: the body gets really cold, teeth chatter, the mind wanders, and the person may stagger around disorientated. If this happens it is important to wrap the person up and keep them warm until they recover.

Method when using a hand-held shower head

- Take your normal shower, nice and warm (not too hot), ensure your body is warm.
- Next, turn the tap to cold and using the hand-held shower move quickly through the routine, covering all areas of the body.

- Run the cold water up your right leg to your right hip, then up your left leg to left hip.
- Bring the cold water up your right arm to your right armpit then do the same with the left arm.
- Next, bring the cold shower all the way from your right foot to the stomach area, chest and neck.
- Quickly do your face and bring the water down your back, buttocks, legs and feet.
- Breathe deeply and scream and yell loudly if it helps! (Screaming and yelling is good for you as it supplies more oxygen to the tissues and is sound therapy as well!). Singing is even better as the sound vibration gets carried by the energy of the water.
- This cold session should only take about 20 seconds.
- Afterwards, turn the tap back to warm and warm up once more if so desired. You may feel a tingling sensation and the colour may rise in your skin.
- You may choose to repeat the cold session for another 20 seconds.
- Finally, turn off the shower and dry yourself vigorously.
- Ensure you dress warmly and move around until your body is nice and warm.
- You will now be ready to face the day or whatever the evening brings!

This cold-water dash is great for fatigue - especially when waking up tired, or after a long day at work, or at the end of the day when you need to freshen up for an evening out. If you are prone to infections, depressive moods, insomnia, general minor circulation problems, or coldness of the hands and feet do try this cold shower regime.

If you live in an isolated area (without neighbours peering over the fence) you may try rolling around on dew covered grass – this is very refreshing!

A great way to start the day (if you are fortunate enough to live in a cold place where there is frost-covered grass in winter) is to run around barefoot on frosty grass - afterwards your feet will glow and be quite warm. Hot saunas and snow go well together.

Ice and cold water

Ice has many uses particularly for pain, muscle tightness, prevention of bruising after an injury, and for fever.

Types of Applications:

- Backache and muscle pains:
  An ice pack for 2 minutes followed by a hot pack for 2 minutes repeated five times every two hours. Always begin with cold and finish with cold.
- Any kind of injury:
  A wet cloth that has iced up in the freezer is useful to wrap around an injured limb, or on any injured part of the body. This will help to prevent bruising and will relieve pain.
- Fever:
  Ice and cold water are both excellent for fever. Wrap blocks of ice in a cloth before applying to the skin. For fever, ice blocks (wrapped in cotton cloth or a small towel) can be placed under the armpits to cool the circulation. Apply for 3 minutes at a time, take a break for 3 minutes and repeat. Cold water packs can be applied under the armpits and over the forehead. Renew when the pack starts to warm and begin with a cold pack again. This treatment is particularly good for babies and children with a high fever. A high temperature is nature's way to destroy harmful bacteria in the body but if the temperature rises too high (over 104 degrees F) it can become a problem especially with babies and children because they may suddenly have a convulsion and fit. Therefore, it is important to keep the body temperature at a level where it is effective yet does not cause a problem.
- Headache:
- Ice or cold water applied to forehead or back of the head where the skull joins the neck.
- Haemorrhoids:
  Ice can be wrapped in a cotton bag and applied to the congested, painful, or bleeding area for up to 20 minutes for relief.

A word of warning – always take care when using ice as it can burn if kept on the skin for too long. Keep checking the area and if at all concerned just use a cold-water pack rather than ice.

Footbath

A footbath is a great way to revive cold or tired feet, or to treat disorders such as headache, migraine, low or high blood pressure, colds and flu, sinusitis, and insomnia.

Method:

- Fill two buckets with cold water.
- Fill another two buckets with warm water, about 38 degrees C. - not too hot, and not too cold.
- A teaspoonful of mustard powder can be added to the warm water for tired and cold feet. Add 3 dessertspoons of mustard powder for cases of headache, migraine, low or high blood pressure, congestion in the head with sinusitis, a cold, or fever.
- Sit on a seat between the hot and the cold buckets.
- Place your feet in the buckets of warm water.
- Remain there for 5 minutes.
- Then place your feet in the buckets with cold water for 10 seconds only.
- Next, place your feet back in the buckets with warm water and stay there for another 5 minutes.
- Again, repeat with feet in the cold water for 10 seconds only.
- Continue this procedure four to six times.
- Dry feet and put on warm socks.
- Walk around for at least 5 minutes to get the best result from this treatment.

Exercise in Water

Any kind of exercise is generally easier to do in water, particularly when there is restricted movement of muscles and joints. Spa and mineral pools are relaxing and therapeutic. Swimming or walking in a pool or dancing to music in water is a great fun way to exercise.

Water as Steam

One of the most effective ways to use water as steam is as an inhalation. An inhalation is useful for colds, influenza, sinusitis, bronchitis, pneumonia, headache, anxiety, and depression or for acne and facial treatments.

Method:

- Bring water to a bubbly boil.
- Pour the boiling water over an herb or a few drops of an essential oil in a basin.
- Cover the head with a towel and keep the face as close as possible to the steam in the basin.
- Inhale slowly and deeply through the nose and mouth.
- Add more boiling water to the basin as the steam diminishes.
- Useful herbs and essential oils to use are Rosemary, Lavender, Eucalyptus, Tea Tree, Orange or Lemon. Essential oils are stronger than herbs and you will only require about 3 drops of an essential oil.

Room Steamer or Infuser

A room steamer can be useful to infuse an herb or essential oil into a room. The reason may be to eliminate bacteria (use Tea Tree, Eucalyptus, or Citrus), or to improve a work or study environment (use Sage, Rosemary, Lavender). Add chosen essential oil to water and bring it to the boil. Allow the steam to infuse throughout the room.

Enema

An enema will cleanse the lower bowel, improve fluid flow in arteries, veins, lymph, and assist in cleansing the liver. It may be administered for constipation, as a plain soap or water enema to the lower bowel. A coffee enema may be administered for a specific purpose, it will have a more stimulating effect on the circulation and it may reach further into the bowel.

Method:

- Plastic disposable enema bags are available which may be purchased empty or filled with fluid. Alternatively, a purpose built enema can, or a hot water bottle can be used (with tube inserted).

- Have a hook or place where the apparatus (with string) can be hung so that it is situated above the body. The fluid must be situated higher than the body to allow the fluid to drain into the bowel.
- A string or handle to hang the apparatus, and a tube with a stopper tap at the other end closer to the body in easy reach to administer the fluid.
- It is advisable to be close to a toilet.
- Ensure stopper on the tap is closed.
- Fill container with water or one teaspoonful of black coffee added to the water.
- Hang the container in a suitable place near where the enema will be administered about one meter above the body.
- Lie comfortably on the right side with the buttock slightly elevated on a cushion.
- Using a little soap, or lubricant, insert the tube into the anus as far as comfortable. Never force the tube, it is a gentle procedure.
- Release the stopper tap slowly to allow the water to flow through the tube into the rectum and large bowel.
- If at any time you feel the urge to defaecate, stop the water and relax until the urge is reduced. Do not end the procedure at this stage. When the urge has passed continue to slowly release water until the full volume is discharged if possible.
- Turn the body to lie flat on your back.
- After about two minutes turn to the left side.
- Next lie flat on your back again.
- Carefully massage the bowel from right to left to help the water move along the bowel as far as possible.
- Hold the water as long as possible then evacuate the bowel contents into the toilet.

Baths

A household bath can be a very relaxing place to be.

- Add up to a cupful of Epsom salts and/or a cupful of sea salt or Himalayan salt to enhance a bath and it will be be therapeutic.

Epsom salt is the mineral magnesium sulphate and when absorbed through the skin from a bath it will encourage the body to relax. Epsom salts can draw impurities out through the skin too and is good to bring boils to a head.

- Add energy to the bath with your favourite essential oil (see Chapter Ten Aromatherapy).
- Add fresh twigs and flowers of rosemary or lavender. Rose petals or jasmine flowers are beautiful scents to add to the bath too.
- For fevers, or when the skin is hot and red (unbroken), for example, sunburn, rash, or chickenpox, add ½ cup of Baking Soda (Soda Bicarbonate) to the bath water. Baking Soda will soothe a burning skin. After the bath a paste of water and Baking Soda applied to the skin can be helpful to stop itching and burning.

Holy Water

Water also has a spiritual significance such as the use of water in baptism and use of 'holy water' as a blessing in other religious rituals.

Conclusion

Hydrotherapy - drinking water, hot and cold showers, packs of ice cold and hot water, footbaths, exercise in water, steam, enemas, bathing, and applying water by any method is related to cleansing, healing, and reinvigorating the body.

On a physical and spiritual note without a doubt all good clean water is a blessing, pure, holy, and a gift from God. The message of water is love and gratitude so let's be thankful for water and return to it love and gratitude!

The world is linked together by love and gratitude." Emoto 2001[41]

CHAPTER FIVE

Fasting and Minerals

Before beginning a fast it is a good idea to start balancing minerals in the body. Minerals are extremely important for normal structure and function of the physical body. Drinking green vegetable juices and pure fruit juices can help to provide minerals during a fast. Alternatively, take tissue salts, sea salt, Himalayan salt, or kelp during a fast. Tissue salts can provide specific mineral nutrition to the cells and these will be discussed in more detail after the section on fasting.

Why fast? What is fasting? How do we fast?

Fasting can have different meanings for different people. For many people fasting is a natural part of their way of life: this can be as a spiritual exercise, a health-related practice, or both.

Fasting for Health

From a physical viewpoint, fasting allows the digestive and other body organs to rest. When the digestive organs are not processing food, energy is used to clear accumulated toxic material from the body, and to cleanse and renew body cells. Fasting helps to eliminate disease and even cancer cells have been known to be starved and controlled or destroyed through fasting. Recent research indicates that, after a five day fast, new stem cells are generated that have the ability to regenerate body cells and tissues. Also, a person can partake of their own urine during a fast and this acts as an individual homeopathic remedy (starting with a teaspoonful).

In some world religions (for example, Christianity, Islam, and Buddhism) fasting is considered a spiritual exercise whereby fasting and prayer go together. When a person fasts as a spiritual exercise, it is to cease eating food and sometimes to stop drinking fluid also. The length of a spiritual fast varies, for example, it may be every day from sunrise to sunset for a specified time (six weeks), or it may be during a certain month of the year, during a religious celebration, once a month for 24 hours, seven days or longer, or for a specific purpose. Sometimes water only is taken during a religious or spiritual fast.

Total mind and body focus during a spiritual fast is generally upon 'S' (Spirit, God, Yahweh, Jehovah). Fasting as a spiritual exercise is sometimes carried out in total silence – either alone or with a group. Common practices during this time are reading scripture or appropriate literature, listening to the spoken word or music, prayer, meditation, contemplation, and listening for inner guidance. Individuals fasting as a spiritual exercise often use this time to meditate and/or contemplate with gratitude for their life and to clear away mental and emotional problems, or to clarify their vision, renew, and grow in spiritual awareness. Also, this is an opportunity for the individual to reflect about what 'S' means to them in their journey through life and what they might do in the future. This can be a time to refocus on a 'calling' or to listen quietly for guidance in starting something new or changing old life style patterns for something better. Journaling the experience is sometimes a useful exercise. The goal is to return to the world refreshed, invigorated, and full of energy for living anew.

In general, at the beginning of any fast one may experience unpleasant symptoms such as nausea, headache, joint pain, and tiredness, but as the fast continues those symptoms vanish and one begins to feel a lightness of the body, more energy, and clarity of mind. As toxic material is eliminated from the physical body, cells regenerate, and the body experiences a newness of life.

It is always advisable when fasting for wellness to begin with a 24 hour fast. Start at mid-day one day and enjoy your last meal. Then drink only fluid until midday next day. Break the fast with a small salad. By sleeping during this time it is easier to do without food. This can become a regular once a week, or once a month, event before progressing to a longer fast. After completing a few 24-hour fasts try a seven day fast. Next, try a fourteen day fast. Work out what suits you best - maybe try several short fasts in a year, or, maybe one long fast perhaps at a retreat center.[42]

Mineral drinks are important throughout a seven day (and longer) fast. These can be made from juiced cucumber, carrot, beetroot or other vegetables and/or apple and lemon juice. To each glassful of mineral drink add a little ginger, turmeric, and a dash of cayenne pepper. Ginger, turmeric, and cayenne are excellent detoxifiers and help with the elimination of toxins from the body. Drink plenty of filtered water too. To every glass of water add a pinch of Himalayan salt (for minerals). Slowly drink one glass of vegetable juice every 2 hours and drink water in between times. An alternative to vegetable juices on a short fast are fruit juices, particularly grape juice, again taken every two hours. Concentrated vegetable and fruit juices can be diluted 50/50 with pure water.

Hunger is common during the first two days into a fast after which hunger generally disappears. Not having to take time out to prepare food and eat it is often a treat and can be one of the most enjoyable aspects of a fast for many.

Some people like to cleanse the lower colon with an enema each day while taking a fast, but this is not altogether necessary if bowel movements have been regular. There are instructions for self-administering an enema in the water section (Chapter 4).

Remember, if you experience headaches, stomach cramps, joint pains, or some other unpleasant symptom this is because the body is starting to clear away toxic material at a deep cellular level. This is a normal part of the healing process. Keep drinking plenty of water, walk in the fresh air, ensure you get enough exercise to stimulate circulation and assist this elimination process. Walking is an excellent exercise particularly walking in the fresh air by the seaside, in the bush, or just walking around a beautiful garden. It is in these places, where the air is fresh and filled with healthy negative ions that natural healing energy is freely available, supportive, and can be very uplifting. Healing energy is all around us in the natural environment so take time to look around, listen to the healing sounds of nature, and deeply breathe fresh air.

Fasting is a good time to rest, relax, reflect, take gentle exercise, and allow the body to cleanse and heal itself so that it can regenerate. Listening to a motivational speaker, or motivational recordings, or reading motivational or inspiring books, are often useful during a time of fasting. Fasting with a family or group is beneficial when it provides positive support. For some people, rather than quietness and silence, listening to favorite classical or energising music is therapeutic. Dancing and singing to music as exercise is good too.

Regular baths or showers will also assist the cleansing process during a healing fast. Cleansing the skin with a loofah brush will scrub the skin and keep pores clean and better able to assist elimination of toxins through the skin. Adding about two cups of Epsom salts (Magnesium Sulphate) and/or sea salt to your bath will also help. As the body eliminates toxic material, cells begin to regenerate and are revitalized providing new energy. The mind becomes clearer and the body feels lighter and more energetic.

After passing through the phase of no appetite or hunger, there will come a time when you feel hungry again. This is usually the time to break a fast and begin to eat again. If you continue to fast beyond your body needs, or what it is capable of achieving well, the body will move into a stage of starvation! Your body intuitively knows and will tell you when it needs food. Whenever you fast, listen to your body.

When breaking a fast it is important, in the beginning, not to indulge in too much food. Always eat small amounts of food for the first few meals. Give yourself one day to slowly return to normal meals. A suggestion is to start breaking the fast with a grated apple followed by a small raw salad then move into larger meals as you return to normal eating patterns. After a very long fast (e.g. a ten day fast) take at least three days to return to regular eating. It is very important to have raw salad foods for your first meal, and not too many mixtures. The effect of this type of food is to sweep the colon clean and get it back to work without using too much energy. Also, this kind of food is much easier on the digestive system as it begins to work normally after the fast. Broths are excellent before returning to normal eating patterns.

Get into the habit of chewing food well. Chewing food well enables you to be satisfied with less food than if you were to eat quickly and it also aids the digestive processes. It has been said that chewing food thoroughly adds years to your life. Rather than swallowing half chewed food (which is hard to digest) chewing food well enables it to be mixed with saliva and when swallowed it provides the right texture for the stomach to continue the process of digestion.

Sometimes it is necessary for an individual to continue working a regular job and this is fine, one can still fast and work.

Fasting is individual: you are unique, so work out the best way to fast for YOU. What works for you may not work for someone else. Start listening to your body. If you feel sick, then that is a good time to fast – stop eating and allow the body to heal itself. Feeling sick may be the body trying to eliminate toxins. If you have high energy before feeling sick, then you are likely to be experiencing a 'healing crisis'– don't rush off and take medicines. Instead allow the body to process whatever it needs to do. Fast, feed your body minerals from fruit and vegetable juices, use home grown herbs as teas (e.g. oat straw, parsley, thyme, sage), and add ginger, or turmeric, or cayenne from the kitchen cupboard to assist the process. Drink plenty of clean WATER.

Unfortunately, most people take medication for a headache when in many cases all the body is doing is crying out for water or for a rest from eating food. Headache is one of the first signs of dehydration or toxins leaving the body cells. Drinking more water is the answer. However, once the body is hydrated, if the headache persists then it may be necessary to seek medical advice.

Fasting can be fun, especially once you gain new energy and the joy of eating returns, and you know that you are successfully reversing disease and regenerating body cells. People who fast regularly are known to live a longer healthier life than those who are forever eating large amounts of food that contribute to obesity, diabetes, or cardiovascular disease.

A word of warning is appropriate here – if you have a serious disorder (e.g. insulin dependent diabetes) consult your medical practitioner before commencing a fast as you may need to be monitored closely during your fast.

Once you become aware of the benefits of fasting you may decide to eat less, for example, two meals a day instead of three. Experiment with eating patterns and find out what works best for you. A large cooked breakfast may satisfy you, or you may choose to miss breakfast and have brunch (breakfast at lunchtime). A main meal may be eaten at mid-day or you may choose to eat a main meal in the evening. Decide what is best for *your* body. However, it may be necessary or best for you to eat three meals at regular times of the day.

Remember it is more important to keep up your fluid intake rather than to eat. Drink plenty of water and you will discover that you probably eat less. Incidentally this is an easy natural way to lose and stabilize weight.

If during a fast you find it difficult to prepare mineral drinks, then you may choose to dissolve specific mineral salts in water according to your needs. I believe the Schuessler system of rectifying cell deficiencies with mineral salts is the best and cheapest way to do it.

Mineral Tissue Salts

Dr Wilhelm Schuessler (1821-1898), a German medical doctor, disillusioned with the results from prescribing medical drugs, compiled a system of healing based upon the minerals which make up the body. These minerals he called tissue salts (often called 'cell salts') which also became known as biochemical or cell salts.

The twelve tissue salts are potentised micro-doses of essential minerals that the human body needs to repair and maintain wellness. They are generally prepared in homeopathic 6x potency and are extremely useful for everyone, particularly babies and children during illness, and adults when fasting. In fact, all the family and even pets can benefit from tissue salts. In a self-help manner, you will be able to treat all symptoms of disease by administering the correct tissue salts.

Tissue salts address mineral deficiencies that are causing *symptoms* of disease. The twelve main tissue salts are:

Calcium Fluoride (Calc. Fluor.)
Calcium Phosphate (Calc. Phos)
Calcium Sulphate (Calc. Sulph.)
Ferrum Phosphate (Ferr. Phos.)
Potassium Chloride (Kali. Mur.)
Potassium Phosphate (Kali. Phos.)
Potassium Sulphate (Kali. Sulph.)
Magnesium Phosphate (Mag. Phos.)
Sodium Chloride (Nat. Mur.)

Sodium Phosphate (Nat. Phos.)
Silicic Oxide (Silica)

Tissue salts are extremely effective, they are rapidly absorbed into body cells because they are finely prepared natural minerals. They are pleasant tasting, generally lactose free, convenient to carry, non-toxic, non-addictive, and safe to use with prescription medicines. The tissue salts are prepared using homeopathic principles, yet unlike standard homeopathy that requires more precise symptom matching, they are suitable for broad, general health complaints, and with a little knowledge are easy to use at home.

By remembering the key symptoms of deficiency for each cell salt it is possible to treat a baby, child, or adult when unwell no matter what the diagnosis or disease may be called.

Tissue salts are dispensed in various forms from dropper-top bottles, powders, or tablets. They can be used as either single tissue salts or mixed in combinations and are conveniently available from pharmacies, health food stores, or on-line stores. The following table shows all tissue salts with their key use, the body component of each tissue salt, and indications when the person may be worse. This key will help you to select the right remedy for the person and to treat deficiencies.

Table 1 Key to Tissue Salts

	Name	Key use	Component of	Worse
1	Calcium Fluoride (Calc. Fluor.)	Deficient tooth enamel. Surface of bones, joints. Hard or cracked skin. Excema. Respiratory infections. Sluggish circulation. Loss of elasticity: varicose veins, haemorrhoids.	Bones & teeth. Elasticity of all body tissues.	Worse in damp, cold, wet weather.
2	Calcium Phosphate (Calc. Phos.)	Poor digestion & assimilation of food. Anaemia. Bone disorders. Respiratory infections	All body tissues, especially teeth and bones. Blood.	Damp, cold weather, and getting wet.

3	3.Calcium Sulphate (Calc. Sulph.)	Spots, pimples, skin disorders, and slow healing wounds. Has a cleansing effect throughout the body. Assists in the removal of waste through the lymphatic system.	Gallbladder (bile) and liver. Dandruff, pimples, boils, shingles, ulcers, abscesses, fistulas, bronchitis, dry eczema, and unhealed cuts	Worse in wet, damp, warm weather, and for physical exertion
4	Ferrum Phosphate (Ferr. Phos.)	Inflammation, redness, throbbing, first stage of respiratory complaints, inflammations, injuries.	All parts of the body, especially red blood cells. Traditional indications: often called the *First Aid Remedy*, early stages of acute disorders, sprains and strains, first stage of fevers. Anaemia. Aids the absorption of iron.	Worse in damp, cold weather, and for getting wet.
5	Potassium Chloride (Kali. Mur.)	Mucous congestion, glandular swellings, coughs, tonsillitis, sore throat, swollen coughs, colds, bronchitis. joints. Disturbances from eating fatty or rich food. Thick, white discharges from skin or mucous membranes. Second stage of inflammation (use after Ferr phos). White-grey coated tongue and light coloured stool	All parts of the body, especially connective tissue. Respiratory system –Glandular or chronic rheumatic swellings. Digestive system.	Worse for motion, physical exertion, and rich foods.
6	Potassium Phosphate (Kali. Phos.)	Nervous tension. Nervous states leading to anxiety, changeable moods, irritability. Tension headaches. Depression, lethargy, exhaustion, Forgetfulness, poor memory. Asthma (stress & emotional) Insomnia. Improves brain function/ exams	Headache, brain fag, nerves, muscles, blood, body fluids.	Worse with worry, stress, exam situations.

7	Potassium Sulphate (Kali Sulph)	Dry scaly skin, dandruff, and skin eruptions, psoriasis. Athlete's foot (tinea). Brittle nails. Late and chronic stage of inflammation. Yellowish or greenish discharge from any mucous membrane or skin surface, yellow slimy tongue. Shifting pains in limbs.	Skin, muscles.	Worse for hot drinks and late afternoon air.
8	Magnesium Phosphate (Mag. Phos.)	Muscle cramps, spasms & muscular twitches. Spasmodic pain or colic, Migraine. Hiccoughs. Sharp twinges of pain. Renal, gastrointestinal, gallbladder, or menstrual colic.	Muscles. Blood cells. Nervous tissue. Bones and teeth.	Worse for cold air, noise, and glare.
9	Sodium Chloride (Nat. Mur.)	Excessive dryness or oedema of tissues, runny nose, loss of smell or taste, salivation, colds with clear discharge and sneezing Disorders of fluid metabolism Excessive fluid or dryness anywhere in the body. Oedema, fluid held in tissues. Craving for salty foods. Headache with constipation. Sadness or depression.	All body fluids and tissues.	Often worse for hot rooms, heat, noise, lying down, and talking.
10	Sodium Phosphate (Nat. Phos.)	Acidity, indigestion or heartburn, rheumatism. An overly acidic system, indigestion or heartburn. Lactic acid build-up in the body, painful muscles and connective tissue, rheumatism. Sciatica. Complaints from fatty food. Acne with greasy skin.	blood cells, muscles, nerve and brain cells, and body fluids.	Worse in thunder storms, mentalexertion, eating fats.

11	Sodium Sulphate (Nat. Sulph.)	Biliousness, liver upsets. Fluid retention, constipation or diarrhoea. Leg ulcers, Poor elimination of metabolic wastes from the body. Rheumatism.	Extracellular fluid.	Often worse for: dampness, lying on left side, pressure
12	Silicic Oxide (Silicea)	Hair, skin and nail problems. Pimples, boils, styes, gum and other abscesses. Excessive perspiration. Lack of strength in connective tissue. Ulcers. Brittle or weak nails. Bunions. Hair loss. Premature ageing.	Component of: skin, hair, nails, muscles, nerves, glands, connective tissue.	Often worse for light, noise, and cold.

CHAPTER SIX

Food and Diet

"Let food be thy Medicine" - Hippocrates

A Word about Diet

Too much emphasis today is placed on food and diet as a requirement for good health and longevity. Let us not dismiss food as unimportant but other factors just as important are often ignored. For example, the healthy elderly Hunza people became a news item and many were keen to know what they ate because their diet was considered to be the answer to their longevity. No doubt food (or the amount of food eaten) did contribute to their longevity but I'm convinced other factors such as a lifetime of work (no retirement there!), social interaction, value of the individual within their cultural group, geographical location, soil conditions and cosmic energies played a big part in sustaining their health and promoting longevity for them. It is easy to say: "This is the answer, eat Hunza food and you will have a long healthy life!" This rarely works due to individual, cultural, environmental, and geographical differences, and varied cosmic energies.

There is not a single diet that suits everyone. Each person needs to work out for themselves what is the best food to eat at any point in time. There are many guidelines to eating but the bottom line is that you need to find what makes you function best and keeps you well.

We are informed that certain types and amounts of foods are required, on a daily basis, to keep us well, i.e., minerals, vitamins, proteins, carbohydrates, and fats. This is mostly true, yet some people defy the dietary recommendations, eat fish and chips, baked beans on toast, bread and butter with a cup of tea, and are still well and live a long, healthy life.

From my experience in clinical practice, using hair as a sample, and epigenetics as a tool, it is possible to analyse individual dietary requirements from a hair sample. Because cells in the body can completely change over a period of three months there may need to be a change to items of diet about every three months. Current epigenetic research indicates many environmental factors cause sickness, or keep us well, and these can be gathered also with the hair sample.

Often, we eat what our parents ate and sometimes this is satisfactory. Culture can play a part in foods we eat but we are still individuals. Since the beginning of time our ancestors evolved and inherited aspects from many different cultures and we know that our genetic imprint has been exposed to different kinds of food. There have been times when our ancestors survived on very little food or relied upon what they grew in gardens or foraged from the land. Animals were caught from the land and bush, or fish came from rivers and the sea. There was no canned, frozen, or processed food available for them to eat so a lot of food was dried, salted, or fermented to preserve it.

Once upon a time we ate foods that were in season. This was good because it gave the body a variety of foods to digest and assimilate and it was always fresh throughout the year. This no doubt fits with the natural evolution of cell changes within the body. Today we can eat anything regardless of season, for example tomatoes. Generally, those tomatoes don't taste the same as ones picked in their normal season. Sometimes vegetables and fruit available in shops are picked before they are ripe or ready to eat. The most nutritious food is organically grown, in season, picked ripe just before it is eaten.

As we add to our shopping basket foods from retail outlets, we are not always aware that food may have been irradiated, grown in an environment of force fertilization, pesticide and fungicide sprays, or may contain all kinds of chemical preservatives. Sometimes apples are waxed to look fresh and shiny to sell and to provide a longer shelf life. These factors can affect our health.

How do we know that we are eating the best food for ourselves? This starts with an awareness of eating fresh nutritious food and knowing from where it comes. Ideally organic food obtained close to the source of production will always be best especially home-grown food picked just before it is eaten. If you are at all concerned about the source of your fruit and vegetables and whether they are likely to have been sprayed with chemicals, soak them in water to which has been added a tablespoonful of apple cider vinegar. Soak for an hour before eating and this will help eliminate toxic residues.

There are ways to determine foods which your body functions best on. One of the quickest ways to know the best foods to eat and foods to avoid is through hair analysis. This is based on epigenetic information specific to the individual. The hair analysis will come at a cost and will be carried out by a practitioner who will take a sample of hair, obtain an analysis through a computer program and data base that provides a comprehensive *Wellness Profile.*[43] The profile will report nutritional deficiencies, food sensitivities, bacterial, viral or fungal infections, environmental considerations, and recommendations for enhancing wellness by following an individual nutritional program.

Other ways to monitor body reaction to food is through either muscle testing or pulse testing. The muscle strength test for intolerances is used by many alternative practitioners as a quick and accurate method to test for food and other allergies. The pulse test was brought to public attention by Dr. Arthur Coca through his book *The Pulse Test for Allergy.*[44] Both tests are easily mastered and can be carried out at home. By testing foods, you will be able to determine which foods suit you best and it will show any sensitivities to particular foods. Just remember if you find that a certain food is not best for you today, it may be alright to eat it in three months' time.

Doing a Muscle test

The muscle test requires help from another person. With your left hand bring your little finger and thumb together and the tips touching. Hold together tightly. Ask your helper to gently try to pull your finger and thumb apart. There is no need to use great force. The idea is to feel the strength at which the finger and thumb is held together. This is the base test that you will monitor the food for testing against. Hold the food for testing in your right hand and bring it close to your body. Alternatively, place a little food on your tongue. Your helper will do the same test again, attempting to draw your finger and thumb apart. The force is consistent with the original test and excessive force is *not* used. If the finger and thumb break free, then the food is probably not good for you at that point in time (weak test). Foods that are good for you will enable your body to maintain a thumb and finger contact (strong test).

Doing a Pulse test

You can easily carry out a pulse test on yourself. Upon rising and before eating anything monitor your radial (wrist) pulse for one minute with your fingers (not your thumb). This will give you your base pulse rate. You are counting heart-beats through the artery that lies alongside the thumb by gently pressing this artery against the bone (radius). You can repeat this test several times during the day (not after strenuous exercise or directly after eating) this will give you an idea of your base pulse rate.

Once you have established your base pulse rate you are ready to start testing foods. It is always preferable to test one food at a time, but this is time consuming and might not be practical. Let's say for example you get up in the morning and are ready to eat an egg on toast for breakfast. Check your pulse before breakfast (let's say it is recorded at 72 beats per minute - your base pulse rate). Then eat your breakfast. Monitor your pulse in 15 minutes (let's say it is now 88). Monitor your pulse again in 30 minutes (let's say pulse is now 90). If after one hour your pulse rate is still recorded at 90 it shows a significant rise from your base pulse rate (up 10 beats or more) and indicates a reaction to your breakfast. You don't know which food is the culprit, so you will now need to start testing each food separately, i.e., toast, butter, egg. Once you have discovered the offending food you should avoid eating it for the next 3 months if possible and then pulse test again. In three months' time you may be able to eat the offending food. Also, you can carry out the pulse test by placing a small amount of a single food on your tongue and holding it for a few seconds, then take your pulse.

It is always best to do the pulse test with a single food, one at a time if possible. Test yourself every three months. Often the same food may test differently. For example, raw food may not affect you, a raw carrot may test with a base pulse rate whereas a cooked carrot may increase your pulse rate, demonstrating a sensitivity to a cooked carrot (or vice versa). However, if the carrot was cooked in a microwave oven, it may not be the carrot but cooking food by this method. The reaction may be due to the effect microwaves have on the carrot, and subsequently the body. If eliminating the suspect food does not stabilize the pulse rate then consider that something in the environment may be the culprit, e.g. dust mites, tree or grass pollen.

Wellness Diary

Another method to work out the best foods to eat is to make a chart or keep a wellness diary. Write down everything you eat, the time, and the amount. At the end of the day make a note of any symptoms you have experienced and if you felt unwell. Also, make a note of when you felt extremely well. See if there are any patterns relating to what you were eating on the days you felt unwell, or well.

If no patterns are discovered related to food, then note further details such as environment factors, for example, the weather, what you were doing, what you were exposed to, what you were wearing, fragrances, people you were with, contact with pets or other animals, social or work situations, did you walk anywhere near chemical sprays, were you exposed to the pollen of trees or flowers? Driving in a motor car? What about emotions (stress, anger, irritation)? and what were you thinking? All these events could be affecting the digestive process and your body metabolism, or the subtle energy field around your physical body.

A Word About Sugar

Sugar definitely needs to be reduced or eliminated from the diet, particularly white refined sugar and processed sugary foods. Excess refined sugar leads to many kinds of health-related problems and chronic diseases. Sugar, sugary drinks, and foods full of sugar are probably doing more damage to people's health than any other product. Where sugar has been introduced into a culture the population experiences tooth decay, obesity and a high incidence of diabetes.

One of the growing trends within the western world, especially the Pacific Islands and New Zealand is chronic disease associated with obesity.

If you crave sugar then you probably need to add more protein, oil, or fat into your diet. Rather than a sweet candy bar, try a handful of nuts or a spoonful of coconut oil. Nuts are nutritious and will sustain blood sugar and energy longer than a candy bar. Read labels on packaged foods and if sugar is listed as one of the first three ingredients avoid that item. Artificial sweeteners are chemicals. Stevia is a natural sweetener.

Excess food

In western OECD countries where there is an overabundance of processed food obesity is becoming a major problem. Associated with obesity are risks for diabetes and heart diseases. Consumption of food can become a health problem. How frequently you eat in the day, what you eat, and how much you eat, may need to be studied if you are overweight. If you are unwell, underweight, or overweight, then experiment with what you eat and the amount of food you eat. Adjustments may need to be made for body size, age and activity level.

Some of the longest-lived people on earth, the Japanese Okinawans, have a saying "hara hachibu" which means eating until one is 80% full. This secret is known to other cultures too. Chewing food well and eating slowly also prevents one eating too much. If food is eaten fast, one is likely to eat more than the body actually needs and abdominal discomfort may result after a meal. The stomach is no larger than the size of your fist so be careful about how much goes into it and how fast you fill it. Some people survive and are healthy and well on very little food.

By drinking water between meals, rather than eating snacks, often the craving for food disappears! Drinking water is an excellent way to help reduce low-density lipoprotein (bad cholesterol), reduce weight, balance hormones, and regenerate cells.

Diet is individual

I do not believe that one diet fits all as far as food and eating is concerned. Work out what suits you best, what makes you function well, and stick to it until you intuitively know that you need to make a change to eating something different. As mentioned, every three months is a good time to do a self-assessment and make some changes to your diet if necessary. If possible, go with the natural seasons of summer, autumn, winter, and spring; and then eat foods that are fresh and appropriate for that particular season. Eventually you will learn the foods on which you function best.

Dr Peter d'Adamo studied people and the relationship of their blood type to the foods they were eating. He discovered that if a person ate the recommended foods that were right for their specific blood type, he/she could be well and experience excellent health.[45] In clinical practice, I discovered too that if people were guided into eating the right foods for their blood type, their state of health improved. You may decide to base your eating according to your blood type. There are four main blood types: A, AB, B, and O. Table 2 provides a simplistic chart to illustrate main food intake differences between the blood groups and a few food sources that are good for each blood group. This is certainly not a complete list of foods and you would be wise to study Dr Peter d'Adamo's book and use the pulse test to set up a chart of your own best foods and foods to avoid.

Table 2: Blood Type Chart

Blood Type	Best type diet	Meat	Fish	Dairy & eggs	Best Nuts & seeds
A	Vegetarian	Avoid red	Small amount	Small amount	Peanuts, pumpkin seeds
B	Mostly vegetarian	OK: Mutton, venison, rabbit	Balance	Best food	None best
AB	Mostly vegetarian	OK: Mutton, turkey, rabbit	Balance	Beneficial	Chestnuts, peanuts, walnuts
O	Mainly meat	OK: Most meats	Good food	Restrict or eliminate	Pumpkin seeds, walnuts
Blood Type	Vegetables (best)	Grains (best)	Beans (best)	Cereals (best)	Fruit (best)
A	Artichokes, beetroot, broccoli, brussel sprouts, Carrots, kale, garlic, ginger, onions, leeks, parsnips, pumpkin, mung bean & alfalfa sprouts	Oat, rice, rye Buckwheat. Rice cakes, essene bread, soya bread	Aduki, black eyed, black beans, pinto, soya, lentils	Buckwheat	Best: Apricot, apple, cherries, figs, raisins, prunes, plums, pineapple

B	Beetroot, broccoli, brussel sprouts, broad beans, cabbage, cauliflower, carrots, kale, parsnips, peppers, parsley, sweet potato, yams.	Oat, rice Brown rice bread, rice cakes. Essene bread, millet bread, wasa bread	Kidney, lima, navy, red, soya	Millet, oats, rice	Bananas, cranberries, grapes, plums
AB	Beetroot, broccoli, cauliflower, celery, cucumber, kale, garlic, parsnip, parsley, sweet potato, sprouts, yams.	Oat, rice, rye Brown rice bread, rice cakes. Gluten free bread. Millet bread. Rye bread, Ryvita. Soya bread. Wasa bread.	Pinto, navy, red, soya	Millet, oats, rice	Cherries, cranberries, gooseberries, grapes, plums
O	Artichokes, broccoli, kale, garlic, onion, leek, parsnips, parsley, pumpkin, sweet potato, seaweed.	None best	Aduki, black-eyed, pinto.	None best	Figs, plums, prunes

There are numerous books about food, eating, diet, and many cookbooks to guide you along a personal pathway to eating well. Read, have fun, stay open-minded and make intelligent decisions that suit *you* and your journey to wellness. Enjoy your food!

Of course, it is more challenging if you decide to become vegetarian or vegan, and everyone else in the household is a meat eater! You may need to be strong and persevere if this is what you function best on. Find a buddy in your community that shares the same beliefs or preferences to act as a support and with whom to share recipes. There are often vegan or vegetarian clubs in some towns. There may be a vegan or vegetarian restaurant where you can sample different foods and meet people. Some church groups are vegetarian, an example is the Seventh Day Adventist Church, who may meet your spiritual needs with fellowship, tasting and sharing vegetarian recipes. I know some men who have taken over the kitchen and learned to cook and prepare meals in order to change the way a family eats.

Mineral deficiencies

As the saying goes, from dust we come to dust we return. The basic structure of the human body is made up of minerals which are also earth elements. These minerals are so important that the body cannot function properly without them.

Symptoms of sickness often relate to deficiencies in the diet and a good starting point is to refer to a nutritional chart that shows symptoms of mineral deficiencies. Vitamins are important for the function of body cells too, but the basic structure of the physical body consists of minerals (see Chapter Five – Tissue Salts).

Macronutrients and Micronutrients

There are seven minerals (macronutrients) that are required by the body in larger quantities than other minerals. These minerals are: calcium, potassium, sodium, chloride (chlorine), magnesium, phosphorus, and sulphur. Other important minerals (micronutrients) or trace elements are required in minute doses, but all are essential for proper development and function of the human body i.e., iron, iodine, silica, manganese, fluorine, zinc, selenium, copper, vanadium, nickel, molybdenum, cobalt, chromium and tin.

In large doses all minerals become poisons to the body. By eating the right foods minerals can be obtained naturally in correct proportions. Sea water contains minerals as well as trace elements so if you live beside the sea a teaspoonful of seawater taken daily will supply adequate minerals and trace elements.

Where there are deficiencies support the body with nutrition first and ensure mineral deficiencies are corrected before rushing off to get drugs or natural medicines. Medicines will often mask symptoms of nutritional deficiencies and, if this is the case, prescribing drugs will not solve the problem. Also, be careful when taking vitamin and mineral supplements that you do not upset the natural and delicate chemical balance of the body. Some supplements (tablets) contain high amounts of vitamins and minerals, much higher than the body actually needs.

Vitamins

Vitamins are required in small amounts by the body and all vitamins can be obtained from foods in the diet if meals are planned carefully. Vitamins are classified as either fat soluble vitamins (A,D,E,K) or water-soluble vitamins (vitamin C and eight complex B vitamins). The fat-soluble vitamins have a diverse range of functions and as a group act as co-enzymes, hormones, and anti-oxidants. Any excess of these fat-soluble vitamins is stored in the liver and fat tissues and an intake of large quantities has been known to cause irreversible harm and damage to body tissues. The water-soluble vitamins act as precursors for co-enzymes, hormones, and antioxidants; any excess is usually excreted from the body.

Some water-soluble vitamins, such as vitamin C are excreted if too much is taken for bodily needs. Therefore, vitamin C is not a problem unless very high doses are taken over a long period of time. Other substances such as high potency multivitamin tablets, or high doses of cod liver oil will build up in cells and tissues and may cause illness. Taking high potency supplements regularly can upset the natural chemical balance within the body and for this reason people are often not functioning to their full capacity when taking supplements.

It is my belief that if you are well there is no need to take supplemental vitamin and mineral pills or potions. The disadvantage of supplements is that each person has different requirements and it is easy to upset the delicate natural chemical balance within the body with high potency supplements. Only resort to supplements if there is a severe deficiency or illness. It is possible to sustain good health through nutrition without the need to take supplements if your food contains adequate minerals and vitamins and lifestyle is balanced. Organically grown mineral rich vegetables and fruit are far superior to any supplement because food has minerals in the correct proportion for human consumption as Mother Nature intended. The advantage of obtaining nutritional requirements from fruit and vegetables if grown in good soil, come to us in a balanced form which are readily and easily digested and assimilated into the body cells. An individually balanced diet, with careful use of herbs and spices, will help you to gain and maintain health and prevent sickness.

Many cultures value broths and have survived on broths during times of famine or crop failure. Broths are full of minerals, whether it is bone broth or vegetable broth. Both are beneficial in sickness and health and will provide readily available minerals for body cells. Bones and green vegetables are rich in calcium and magnesium which are two minerals extremely important for the prevention of numerous diseases.

Proteins

The human body consists of 20% protein. Amino acids are the building blocks for proteins and are essential for the structure and function of the body. Some amino acids can be synthesized in the body and some cannot. These essential amino acids must be, and can be, gained from foods. First-class proteins, which are considered complete proteins, are meats, poultry, fish, and dairy products that contain all the essential amino acids. Second-class proteins, considered incomplete proteins, do not contain all essential amino acids in one food source, but can be gained from a variety of second-class protein foods eaten together. For example, any of the following combinations of second-class proteins can provide a first-class protein: soya beans, chick peas, black beans, lima beans, cereals, nuts, lentils, corn, rice, pasta, and fresh vegetables. There are plenty more vegetable food sources that can be combined to provide a first-class protein. It is important that vegetarians and vegans study food combinations in order to obtain their complete protein sources from their diet.

Protein is necessary for healing wounds and repairing tissues, especially in muscles, bones, skin and hair, as well as for the removal of waste products in connection with metabolism. Protein eaten is broken down in the digestive system into individual amino acids and then reconstructed as new tissue protein through the process of biosynthesis. Problems arise in the body when cells do not receive all essential amino acids. If one or more of the amino acids are deficient the body is weakened in some way.

Unfortunately, other substances enter the human body alongside some proteins such as when chickens have been fed hormones and antibiotics with their food, as well as plant proteins sprayed with pesticides and other chemicals. These things affect human metabolism and weaken the body too.

Fats and Oils

Fats have two important functions in the body: to assist in the absorption of fat soluble vitamins and secondly to supply essential fatty acids that cannot be synthesised by the human body. There is a thin fat (lipid) layer in the membrane around each cell in the body that provides structure and helps protect cells from invasion by bacteria and viruses and any other harmful product. Brain, nerve, and muscle cells need fats to enable them to function well. Fat is also a major source of energy. It satisfies hunger and spares protein. Stored in the body, excess fat is deposited in the tissues and called adipose tissue and can be used when food is scarce. All meats contain fat. Olive, linseed, sunflower, and coconut oil, are good vegetable oils, almond is a good nut oil, and all fish oils are excellent and important in the role of sustaining cellular health. Coconut oil is the most stable at high heat so is good for cooking. Cold pressed oils are better than any oils processed with chemicals or high heat.

Carbohydrates

Carbohydrates are sugars and starchy foods and their main function is to supply readily available energy. Digested complex carbohydrate food releases energy and supplies dietary fiber which adds bulk to waste material in the large bowel. Carbohydrate spares protein because it is used first for energy rather than proteins. Carbohydrates can increase blood sugar very quickly, but also get used fast, then blood sugar decreases quickly. Protein foods raise the blood sugar slowly and keep it steady for a longer length of time than sugar or carbohydrate foods. Carbohydrate spares protein so that protein can be used for other important functions within the body such as growth and repair of cells and tissues.

Carbohydrate foods include bread, sugar, jam, honey, cereals, rice, pasta, semolina, and vegetables.

The Glycaemic Index (GI)

This is a chart that ranges from 1-100. A food's Glycaemic Index indicates the rate at which the carbohydrate in a particular food is broken down into glucose and absorbed from the gut. Foods lower on the chart are better for people with Diabetes and dieters looking to reduce their carbohydrate intake. These foods have higher levels of protein, fat, and fiber. These three compounds slow down the body's ability to process sugar. Dairy and pasta are examples of products low on the GI chart.[46]

Ways to Eat

Eat a balanced diet to be well and discover what is right for you. Don't be afraid to experiment with foods, you may need to try different ways of eating until you are satisfied, function well, and remain healthy.

Listed below are some popular diets in no particular order. There are plenty of books available to expand your reading in any one of these nutritional regimes, as well as recipe books to match the style.

- RawVegan
- Vegan
- Vegetarian
- Plant Based
- Fish
- Carnivore
- Omnivore
- Flexivore

Utilising fresh, nutritional rich food is extremely important if you want to nourish the body properly and sustain health. Diets prescribed by naturopaths generally consist of fresh foods, raw foods, non-processed wholesome foods without chemical additives, organic foods, vegetable and fruit juices. Changing from a carnivore type diet to vegan or vegetarian will reduce levels of Vitamin B12 over time and this problem may need to be addressed by some people. It appears that children born to vegetarian mothers and brought up with this kind of balanced diet do not suffer B12 deficiency.

Fermented Foods

Fermented foods are good for gut health and can be easily made at home.

Sauerkraut

Sauerkraut changes cabbage by lacto-fermentation into a delicious tasty food that contains healthy probiotics. All that is required is a fresh cabbage, salt, and a stone crockpot or glass jar suitable for making the sauerkraut. A jar with stones or marbles in it to fit the mouth of the jar or pot to weigh down the cabbage while it is fermenting is necessary and a cover to keep insects away. Some people like to add caraway seeds to add flavor but this is not necessary.

Method

A one quart jar will take a medium size cabbage and about two tablespoonfuls of salt.

- Wash hands and all jars before starting.
- Chop fresh cabbage and mix with salt.
- Optional - mix in one teaspoonful of caraway seeds.
- Pack cabbage firmly into the jar. Press down each layer as you pack.
- Press cabbage down with jar weighted with stones or marbles.
- Cover with muslin cloth and tie down with a rubber band.
- Over the first 24 hours continue to press cabbage down. Juice will begin to come out of the cabbage and the fermentation process will begin.
- Ensure that the cabbage is always kept below the juice.
- If necessary add a little water (water is not generally needed) to keep cabbage covered with fluid.
- After three days try the sauerkraut for taste. It can be eaten now.
- Most times you will allow the cabbage to ferment further.
- As the cabbage continues to ferment bubbles occur and perhaps a scum will form on the top. This is normal and scum can be scooped off.
- When the taste is to your liking, keep it in the refrigerator.
- It keeps well for several months.

Apple Cider Vinegar.

When apples are in season you can make a supply of Apple Cider Vinegar that will last for a year. A teaspoonful of Apple Cider Vinegar in a glass of water first thing in the morning makes a refreshing start to the day.

Method

A large jar or jars. Plenty of apples (any kind will do).

- Clean hands and jars required.
- Cut up apples – skins, cores and all.
- Fill jar(s) with apples.
- Cover apples with clean water (filtered if possible).
- As with sauerkraut above weight the top of the jar to ensure apples stay underwater.
- Cover jar with muslin cloth.
- Leave and watch the fermentation process.
- Between two and six weeks your Apple Cider Vinegar will be ready.
- Test by smelling – it should have the fresh smell of vinegar.
- Taste – when it tastes right, strain and bottle.

A Word About Seeds

Seeds hold the essence of life within them. Given the right conditions a seed will always grow and go through its cycle of life: sprouting, growing, producing, and finally reproducing through its own seeds.

Today seeds have been interfered with and genetically modified to the extent that some seeds purchased will grow vegetables, but *they will not reproduce* or if they do produce seeds those seeds will be useless. Those seeds will *not* grow vegetables again. According to AgWeb,[47] the "big four" biotech seed companies: Monsanto (now Bayer), DuPont/Pioneer, Syngenta and Dow AgroSciences own 80 percent of the U.S. corn market and 70 percent of the soybean business. They also control more than half the world's seed supply. Considered by some as 'evil global corporates', these companies could gain enough power to eventually control the worlds food sources, allowing fewer choices and demanding higher prices for seeds and food.

Factors that have led to industry domination by a few players in the United States of America include the purchase of smaller seed companies by larger companies and weak antitrust law enforcement. Supreme Court decisions have allowed genetically engineered (GE) crops and other plant materials to be patented, while prohibiting seed saving by farmers. Farmers who have not saved any seeds are now forced to buy fresh seeds every year from the controlling companies.

More than 40 years ago in New Zealand some resourceful people saw what was happening so they started 'seed banks' where seeds could be saved and stored. Several individuals and organisations now have valuable collections of heritage fruit and vegetable seeds collected over the years that they continue to grow from, save seeds, sell, swap, and promote the continued reproduction of seeds. Provided people continue to save seeds New Zealand has a bright future. Many individuals are now saving their own seeds as a means of food security for the future.

Over the years many seed banks have become established across the world where people have gathered some amazing collections of seeds. In some countries these seeds cannot be sold so people gather and have 'seed swap' days where they can swap seeds or give them away. Saved seeds from seed banks *will* reproduce and home gardeners are now encouraged to save their own seeds and reuse them again, and again, each year. The time is rapidly approaching when people will be unable to purchase the type of seeds from retail outlets that will produce viable seeds.

When purchasing seeds, it is advisable to buy them from a seed bank or a reliable source where you know that they have not been interfered with. Always let a plant or two go to seed in your own garden and develop your own bank of seeds for the next year for future generations and to share with others.

Always harvest seeds on a dry sunny day. Seeds from cucumbers or pumpkins can be washed and spread out on paper in the sunshine, or in a dry place, until they are dry. Keep seeds dry in brown paper bags, airtight tins, or glass jars and store them in a cool place until ready to be planted. As you save seeds, you will find that there will be enough to give away thus generations of pure seeds will be passed on. If you don't have a seed swap group in your town, consider starting one.

Sprouted seeds for food

In the kitchen you can sprout seeds in a jar and eat them after a few days. These seeds are full of life and extremely nourishing. Three seeds that are easy to grow and will be ready in a few days are wheat, alfalfa and mung beans. My favorite are mung beans. Ensure seeds are fresh and have not been genetically modified at all otherwise they will not sprout. Be sure the seeds are edible and do not purchase from a garden or farm centre either where seeds have been coated with chemicals to make them grow. The best place to purchase edible seeds is direct from a food store that sells organic products *or* grow your own.

To sprout seeds:

- Place seeds in a glass jar. Seeds will swell to about three times their volume.
- Cover with warm water and leave at lease twelve hours (in a warm place if wintertime).
- Place a muslin cover or steel net over the top of the jar, to stop insects entering the jar and to allow water to drain easily when rinsing the seeds.
- After twelve hours drain off the water through the muslin or net top.
- Rinse the seeds every day with warm water and allow to drain.
- Place the jar in a warm, light place (such as a windowsill).
- Over a few days the seeds will start sprouting.
- The seeds are ready to eat when soft and starting to sprout.
- Start a fresh batch every day (or every second day), for a regular supply.

By the third day the sprouted seeds are usually ready for eating (depending upon the weather). Seeds sprout faster in warm weather. In a hot climate or during the summer season you may need to rinse seeds more than once a day. In a colder climate, seeds will take longer to sprout - maybe four days, but if you keep them in a hot water cupboard or warm place they will sprout more quickly. Eat the seeds as soon as they start sprouting. They are best eaten raw. Once seeds have sprouted to the appropriate size for that seed, keep them in a refrigerator to slow the growing process. If left too long, sprouts will grow green leaves and become bitter. At this stage don't waste them – add them to soups, stews, stir fry vegetables or, plant them in your garden and let them grow to provide you with a fresh supply of seeds.

When wheat seeds become leafy transfer them to a small round pot of soil and let them grow further. Use the freshly growing wheat grass as a 'Biogenic Battery' for meditation.

The Biogenic Battery

Either grow wheat seeds specifically for your biogenic battery or transplant sprouted seeds that have grown too leafy to eat into a pot and allow them to grow further.

Edmond Szekely a follower of the Essene tradition has this to say about the Biogenic Battery:

"We discover every one of the sixteen natural and cosmic forces in the Biogenic Battery… it is a true representation of health as it unites all the forces of sun, water, air, food, earth, and joy…Love is another force which is experienced through tactile contact with the Biogenic Battery. When we hold the grass between our palms during Biogenic Meditation, a tremendous amount of excess energy flows to us from the Biogenic Battery This gift to us of its energy is love - in its most direct and selfless form."[48]

The technique is to sit comfortably with your hands clasped around the wheat grass and meditate in whatever manner it suits you. Close your eyes and let your mind quieten and just be still as you experience the energy of the universe in the growing shoots of wheat grass.

In conclusion

Individual diet and nutrition requires a lot of common sense on the pathway to wellness. Eliminate toxins, drink plenty of clean fresh water, ensure essential nutrients are balanced in the body by eating home grown or organic fruits and vegetables. Work out a diet that suits your individual needs and reassess yourself every three months. Soon you will discover how to sustain your physical body with the right type of food, the manner in which you need to prepare it, the amount you need to eat, as well as any significance in the times of the day (or night) you need to eat in order to function well. Chew food well, don't overeat, in gratitude give thanks for the love and energy that created the food and perhaps gave its life to nourish your body in order for you to attain excellent health.

Finally, as you gain an understanding about your body and what it needs for wellness there will be no need to run hither and thither searching for new diets or nutritional regimes because there will be no better way for you. You will have found what is right for YOU as an *individual* and will no longer need to pay attention to what others are saying or eating. Be the authentic well-nourished person you were meant to be.

*"Only foods provide the exact nutrients the body needs to heal itself...
Each of us is unique, and our nutritional needs differ from person to person."*
Dr Bernard Jensen[49]

CHAPTER SEVEN

Homeopathic Home Remedies

A minute dose of energy medicine works miracles

Homeopathy is an extremely safe form of natural energy medicine that treats the whole person and these remedies are sure and safe. Homeopathic remedies are a means to sustain well-being, to use as *First Aid* and to use for common sicknesses in the home. Like all forms of natural medicine, homeopathic remedies rely on the body's own powers of self-healing. The rationale behind homeopathic medicine will be explained and secondly, a few well tested remedies will be presented that you may want to try. The remedies listed here have stood the test of time and further remedies can be found in William Boericke's popular *Homeopathic Materia Medica with Repertory.*[50]

The founder of Homeopathy was Samuel Hahnemann (1755-1843), a German Physician who became dissatisfied with medical practices of his day. Hahnemann qualified as a medical doctor in 1779 and spent many years trying to support his large family by means other than medicine, i.e., translation and writing. He had strong views about medical practices that prescribed large doses of drugs and the common practice of blood–letting. Lunatics were treated very harshly and given purges, emetics, starved, flogged, and tied up. Hahnemann was concerned about these people and how they were treated. He sought a better way and was an advocate for fresh air, good food, and exercise. He was well in advance of his time as he endeavoured to find something kinder and safer to heal sickness, particularly mental illness.

While doing translation work in 1790 Samuel Hahnemann stumbled across the principle called the 'law of similars'. This law is based on the principle that 'like cures like' which means that a substance that causes certain symptoms in a healthy person could cure a sick person with the same symptoms (no matter what the diagnosis or sickness). Hahnemann experimented successfully on himself with quinine to test his theory and went on to formulate a set of principles for treatment with what he called homeopathic remedies. Hahnemann eventually produced the first homeopathic *Materia Medica*.

His method was to prove substances in large quantities that created symptoms in a healthy person could cure the same symptoms in a sick person when made into homeopathic formulations. The number of remedies listed in the *Homeopathic Material Medica* have increased over time, yet the same remedies used during the time of Samuel Hahnemann are still in use today. The *Materia Medica* is a text with all the information about remedies that have stood the test of time for treating people in a safe, natural, and drugless manner.

To explain a little further; the patient's symptoms are matched with the same symptoms that a substance in its raw state is capable of producing in a healthy person. For example, the symptoms of arsenic poisoning are abdominal pain, vomiting, continual thirst, prostration, and diarrhoea. Some of these symptoms occur with dysentery, therefore arsenic in its homeopathic form can be used to treat dysentery. Allium Cepa (red onion) in its raw state will cause tears to well, a watery discharge to run from the nose, and even sneezing to occur, therefore it is a useful homeopathic remedy for the first stages of a common cold.

All homeopathic remedies are chosen because of their proven power to produce in a healthy person, symptoms similar to those manifested in the sick person. The word homeopathy is taken from two Greek words homeo - like or similar, and pathos - feeling or suffering. It is a system of medicine that has fixed principles from which to work and remedies that do not drug the body.

A professional homeopath when taking a case will inquire into and record all possible facts concerning the signs and symptoms of the whole person, from the mind to the skin. Of these, the mind symptoms and any strange or unusual symptoms are important. After the client has related all details about pain, times of aggravation, likes and dislikes, relationship to anything hot or cold, wet or dry weather etc., it is possible to build up a picture of the whole person and then determine the individual remedy for that particular person. It is considered both an art and a science to select the correct homeopathic remedy. Selecting a wrong remedy will do no harm (unless prescribed in an extremely high potency) and will not be effective either. Often the reason why homeopathy lost popularity for treating sickness is because the wrong remedy was selected for the persons symptoms.

Homeopathic Remedies

Homeopathic remedies are made from plant, animal, and mineral extracts, they are diluted in varying degrees, then succussed, to form a vibrational, energy medicine. Ironically, the more dilute the remedies become and the further they are succussed (shaken) the more potent or powerful and effectively they work. The making of remedies is very precise. For remedies made from soluble substances, such as animal or plant extracts, the raw material is dissolved in an alcohol/water mixture that contains approximately 90 per cent pure alcohol and 10 per cent distilled water (this can vary with different substances). This mixture is left to stand for 2-4 weeks, shaken occasionally and then strained through a press. The resulting liquid is known as the mother tincture. Insoluble substances (gold, calcium carbonate etc.) need to be made soluble by a process known as trituration, in which they are ground continually until they become soluble. Then they are diluted and used in the same way as the soluble substances.

Samuel Hahnemann first began applying the *Law of Similars* in his medical practice and then began to experiment with the size of the dose to see how little of the substance would still effect a healing response. It took him years but eventually he found a method of diluting (and succussing) the substance to a minimum while the potential to cure was magnified. He called this process 'potentization'.

Making of a remedy

If the medicine is soluble it is diluted in water or alcohol according to a decimal or centesimal scale and the mixture is shaken vigorously by striking the bottle against a firm surface (succussed). If the medicine is insoluble it is finely ground, or triturated, and mixed with powdered lactose (milk sugar). One part of the diluted medicine is then diluted again in the same manner until the correct strength is achieved.

Potentization is different from simple dilution. Homeopaths have found that the medicines do not work if they are simply diluted repeatedly without vigorous shaking or if they are just diluted in vast amounts of liquid. Nor do the medicines work if they are only vigorously shaken. *It is the combined process of dilution and shaking that makes the medicine effective.*

To produce different potencies, the mother tincture is diluted in an alcohol/water mixture according to one of the two most commonly used scales:

Decimal scale (x). This is a one in ten scale dilution, 1:10.

Centesimal scale (c) This is one in a hundred scale dilution, 1:100.

Between each stage of dilution, the diluted tincture is succussed.

To produce a 1x potency of a remedy one drop of the mother tincture is added to 9 drops of an alcohol/water mixture and succussed. To produce 2x potency remedy one drop of the 2x mixture is added to 9 drops of alcohol/water mixture and succussed. For a 3x potency remedy one drop of 2x to 9 drops of alcohol/water mixture and succussed, and so forth. After the 6x potency remedy has been made there is no trace of the original substance, only the *vibrational energy* of the substance remains. The number of a homeopathic remedy shows how many times it has been diluted and succussed to produce its potency. The most common potency available at retail outlets is either 6x or 30x, which are also the safest and most effective doses for home use.

Storing remedies

It is best to keep your homeopathic remedies out of direct sunlight and away from strong odours as well as in a cool place. Do not store them in a bathroom cupboard with soap or essential oils, or on a hot kitchen shelf as these things may affect the remedies and reduce or nullify the effectiveness of their action.

Dosage

Always use the smallest amount of the indicated remedy to produce the desired effect. It is always advisable to begin with a low potency remedy (3x, 6x, or 30x)

Chronic (long standing) diseases with mental symptoms may require higher potencies (100x, 1000x, or 1M). The optimal dose is one which does not cause a reaction yet heals. The remedy must be suited to the needs of the *individual*. If the potency is too low, no improvement will occur in the person's condition. If the potency selected is too high, the entire symptom picture may be made worse, but no new or unusual manifestations may appear. Such an increase in the symptoms is termed an aggravation and care should be taken to guard against it. High doses may aggravate the condition. The inability to select with accuracy the correct dose for the individual has accounted for many failures with homeopathic medicine.

As a general rule – the potency to be given will be governed by the following considerations.

1. Low potencies 1x, 3x, are usually given in chronic pathological states.
2. Medium potencies 6x, 12x, 30x are usually given for acute disorders.
3. High potencies 100x upwards are given for mental symptoms.

When all individual symptoms are matched perfectly to the remedy then the higher potencies will work miracles.

Frequency of dose

In acute disorders the indicated remedy can be given two or three times a day (generally a low potency 6x to 30x). In acute disorders it can be taken up to every 10 minutes, until improvement in the condition commences, then the dosage is stopped, and the sick person observed. If the improvement lapses, then another dose is given.

In chronic disorders, or when a higher potency is indicated, the dose is given sometimes, once a week, or once a month, or at even longer intervals. Always remember, when the individual has reacted well to the indicated remedy, and their condition has improved, the dose should be reduced at once (or even stopped) and the medicine allowed to continue its action.

The Golden Rule in Homeopathy

Stop all medicine as soon as improvement has set in and wait. If the person should slip back, then repeat the dose, but **so long as improvement**

is taking place do not repeat or take another remedy. It is usual to use one remedy at a time.

Other Rules

The rule about taking a homeopathic remedy in a 'clean mouth' doesn't seem to be as important as it used to be, yet if possible abide by the ruling. People were always instructed to avoid taking coffee, drugs, smoking or cleaning their teeth with flavoured toothpaste prior to taking the remedy. In today's hustle and bustle and pace of life, this may be almost impossible, but rinsing the mouth is a good idea before taking a remedy. Since homeopathic remedies are vibrational remedies, the individual is still getting the benefit and the remedy still works. The list of remedies here are selected as the best remedies for use as First Aid remedies and remedies for common conditions at home.

In deep-seated chronic conditions it is more appropriate to take a very detailed case history and then match those symptoms with the remedies in a *Materia Medica*. This can be complicated and time consuming and requires an in-depth knowledge of all the homeopathic laws, the selection process, disease classification, and modalities, as well as knowledge about use of the *Materia Medica*. In chronic conditions it is best to seek the advice of a qualified homeopath. Self-help information provided here does not expand into further detail so none of these laws will be explained. The aim is to provide you with a working and practical knowledge of a few common and effective remedies that you can use at home to treat common ailments.

It is worth noting that it was Hahnemann's teaching that the *removal of the cause* was the first step in the proper method of cure. Today the same advice applies. That may mean a surgical procedure, a change of diet, the removal of irritating sprays and poisonous substances, a change of environment, removal of anything and everything so the person is placed in the best possible situation for a complete cure. He also believed that disturbances in the vital force from outside influences of various kinds could result in disease. Therefore, the aim of homeopathic medicines is to stimulate the individual's vital force to bring about healing.

The list of homeopathic remedies selected here can be administered for self-help at home quite safely. Build up your medicine box as you try them out. Be careful about how and why you choose a remedy and remember to stop when healing begins and let the vital energy of the body finish the work.

Key signs and symptoms are given for each remedy as well as any peculiar traits. The most common symptoms are in *italics*.

Aconite

Aconite is a remedy for the beginning stage of acute complaints. Useful in conditions brought on by exposure to a draught or cold wind. It is indicated by the *sudden onset of sharp symptoms*. The person is restless and agitated and their face may express *anxiety, fear or panic*; fear of death. The face may be pale or flushed. *Skin dry and burning*. It can be used for a cold or fever where there is extreme thirst for cold water. Sickness coming on suddenly *before midnight*, after exposure to a draught of cold air, a cold temperature, or dry winds. Examples are *sudden violent headache*, croup, cough, head cold, and sore throat. A child often complains of earache or sore throat at bedtime. An adult may be sleepless from mental agitation or insomnia after a shock or fright. Toothache.

Allium Cepa

Allium Cepa (red onion) is the best remedy for the *beginning of a cold* where there is *frequent sneezing and a watery discharge* that irritates the nose and eyes stream tears. These symptoms are similar to a healthy person peeling onions. Allium Cepa is also useful for *hay fever*, sneezing, and a cough causing pain and sharp tearing sensation in the throat. The person is *worse in a warm room* and feels better in the open air and a cold room.

Apis Mellifica

Apis mellifica is the remedy for bee stings and insect bites with *swelling, itching. and redness*. Any symptoms similar in nature to a bee sting, from whatever cause, can be treated with apis. Typical symptoms are *stinging, burning pains*, puffy swellings which may be around the face, eyelids, eyes, mouth, or in the throat (with difficult breathing). There is little thirst and little urine. The person is worse from heat, touch, pressure, after sleeping, and in a closed heated room. The person is better from cold applications, motion, in the open air, and removing clothing or bed covers.

Arnica

Arnica is a very versatile remedy. This remedy is top of my list – if you purchase no other remedy then this one is useful to always have on hand. Use it in all *shock situations:* it can be taken when you receive bad news and suffer emotional shock. Administer *after falls, injuries,* concussion, *bruising,* black eye, *surgery, dental extractions, and childbirth.* Give immediately after a blow, fall or physical shock and it will counteract ill effects. Arnica diminishes and *alleviates pain.* It promotes speedy healing. It can be used for sore muscles after overexertion, and for sprains around joints. It can be used for measles and influenza where muscles and joints are sore. Administer for *fatigue* and overwork. Do *not* take large amounts of arnica for any length of time before surgery, because prolonged use may cause excessive bleeding during surgery.

Belladonna

Belladonna is a remedy used for *sudden onset* of symptoms. Key symptoms are restlessness, *red face, violent throbbing headache with heat, as well as colds (sudden sore raw throat), influenza, cough, fever, earache* and red face. A typical symptom is sudden onset of fever, especially in children. Skin dry and hot to the touch, eyes red, sensitive to the light, pupils dilated. *Throbbing pain*, congestive headaches. Earache seems to appear especially in the right ear, after getting the head cold or wet. Sunstroke with redness and pounding pulse needs this remedy. *Whooping cough* responds well to belladonna.

Bryonia

Bryonia acts on all *serous membranes* and the *organs* they contain as well as *around joints. Swollen, hot, shiny joints.* The general character of pain is a *stitching, tearing pain: worse by motion, better at rest. Headaches* that are worse from movement. *Vertigo* and giddiness from raising the head. Colds and other complaints coming on in warm weather. Hard *dry cough, pleurisy. Acute illness*, with thirst for long drinks at frequent intervals. Motion, touch and pressure aggravate the pain. *Constipation* with large, dry and hard stools. The person is usually irritable, and complaints may be brought on by anger. Children dislike being carried or raised and want things, which are refused when offered. Physical weakness with apathy. Wants to be quiet and left alone.

Calcarea Carbonica

Calcarea Carbonica is a remedy suited to *fat, flabby children, who sweat at night,* and take cold easily. *Teeth are slow to show, and faulty teeth* often develop. Children with *knock-knees or bowlegs* and are late to walk. Young girls with *period problems* - either profuse or long lasting, with anaemia, or perhaps late and scanty. *Obese adults.* Chilly and *bad circulation* - takes cold easily. *Pituitary and thyroid dysfunction.* A peculiarity is a craving for eggs, sweets, and an aversion to milk.

Cantharis

Cantharis symptoms are typically a *burning pain* which is characteristic in *cystitis* when there is frequent, burning, *painful urination* with an intolerable urge to pass urine. *Burns and scalds* with rawness and smarting. Cantharis can be used internally or externally for burns (with or without formation of blisters) on the skin. Use for any symptoms causing burning sensations e.g., *burning sensation on the soles of feet at night.*

Carbo Vegetabilis

Carbo vegetabilis is the remedy for *sudden collapse* from any cause. Collapse or other ill effects from an *exhausting* illness e.g., measles, whooping cough, typhoid. Patient looks grey, cold sweat, gasps for air. Limbs cold, *cold, clammy and bluish skin,* cold knees in bed. Effects of *alcoholism.* Injury, or haemorrhage. All foods disagree, *excessive flatulence, abdomen distended, sour belching, regurgitation of food and burning sensation* in the throat. The person has an aversion to milk and meat.

Chamomilla

Chamomilla is one of the best remedies for *teething babies and children* who are fractious, excitable, asking for things then throwing them away. Child wants to be carried all the time. *One cheek hot,* the other pale and cold. *Diarrhoea,* especially with teething, *stools acrid, greenish colour.* Adults with a similar temperament as above. Insomnia – tired and sleepy but can't sleep, especially after a mental upset. *Sensitive to pain* – patient says unable to endure pain. *Toothache and earache* with severe pain. *Labour pains* are erratic and distressing. Worse from warmth. Thirsty.

Gelsemium

Gelsemium is the best remedy for a typical attack of *influenza* – shivers up and down the back, aching in back and limbs, tight headache, half-closed eyes, dim vision and sore eyeballs. Summer colds with mild fever. Watery discharge from nose with much sneezing. *Dry cough with sore throat. Tiredness and aching of whole body.* Limbs, head, eyelids feel heavy. *Chilled with shivers* up and down the back. *Headache* as if a band around the head. Dizziness, drowsiness, trembling, and dullness. Often symptoms develop several days after exposure. Often no thirst even with fever. Worse from damp weather, tobacco smoking. Better from open air, continued motion, bending forward

Hypericum

The key for hypericum is *injuries to nerves.* Hypericum heals injured parts rich in nerves, such as the fingertips and toes. It is also beneficial for tailbone injuries, even old ones. Other indications for hypericum are puncture wounds from nails, bites, and splinters. *Crushed injuries to finger or toe nails.* Pain shoots upward from the wound, especially up the limbs, or in the case of the spine, pain shoots up and down. *Dental surgery, including root canal work or tooth extraction. Eye injuries.* Relieves *pain after an operation.* Speeds healing of jagged cuts. Worse from dampness, fog, touch, cold.

Ipecacuanha

Persistent nausea and vomiting is the chief guiding symptom for ipecacuanha. Nausea not relieved by vomiting. Vomiting during pregnancy. *Asthma* attack. *Incessant violent cough* with every breath. Pale, cold sweaty with weak pulse. Worse from motion, lying down, dry weather.

Ledum

Ledum is the remedy for *puncture wounds from sharp pointed objects* such as needles, nails, splinters. One of the best remedies to take after insect stings (especially mosquito). Ledum will prevent and treat *tetanus* and is useful for *animal bites* and scratches. Worse from warm applications, heat, especially in bed at night. Injured parts are relieved by cold applications.

Nux Vomica

Nux vomica is the best remedy for *bad effects of drink, food, and drugs*, e.g., coffee, alcoholic beverages, tobacco, highly seasoned spicy foods, and drugs. It is also a remedy to soothe an *irritable*, nervous system, and for people who are *hypersensitive, angry,* and over impressionable. For people who are hypersensitive to noise, touch, light, odours, dry weather, drafts and cold. *Constipation* with frequent and ineffectual urging to pass faeces. *Travel sickness. Nausea with headache,* retching. Worse in early morning, from mental exertion, and cold open air. Better from rest, strong pressure, warmth, and in the evening.

Pulsatilla

This is pre-eminently a remedy for *childhood illnesses and females* (especially for mild, gentle yielding disposition). *Sensitive, weepy symptoms,* desires attention and sympathy. *Changeable symptoms. Stomach upsets from rich foods.* Aversion to fats. Insomnia from reoccurring thoughts. Mucous membrane affected, discharges thick, bland, yellowish green. To dry up mother's milk when no longer needed. Helpful in childhood illness e.g. *measles, mumps and chickenpox.* Dryness of mouth with lack of thirst. Unbearable pain. Worse from rich fatty foods, after eating, lying on left or painless side and in a warm room. *Worse heat* and hot fluids. Better from motion, fresh open air, cold food and drinks although not thirsty.

Rhus Toxicodendron

Rhus toxicodendron is for *tendons, muscle sheaths* and indicated when *joints* are painful tender, and stiff. *Arthritis* relieved by damp. Useful after injury or surgery on tendons. *Sciatica. Sharp pains.* Triangular red tip to the tongue. *Chicken Pox* and *shingles. Cellulitis and infections* such as boils and carbuncles in the early stages. Septicaemia. Usually worse in wet and rainy weather.

Sepia

Sepia is pre-eminently *a female remedy* - it acts upon the uterus, ovaries and vagina. Premenstrual syndromes when menstruation painful or heavy. Menses can be scanty, with headache and acne on the face. *Emotional and physical symptoms* during and after *pregnancy. Morning sickness of pregnancy -* nausea from thought or sight of food. *Hot flushes* during *menopause* and alopecia (falling hair) at menopause. *Circulatory problems* (for hot and cold flushes and varicose veins). Persons inclined to be *depressed, weeps easily,* does not seek sympathy, also fear of being alone. Indifference to loved ones. Worse from rest, cold, and before thunder. Better from walking fast, warmth.

Sulphur

Sulphur has an affinity for the *skin. Hot, burning, itching skin,* red lips and eyelids. Uncomfortable when standing. *Talks, jerks and twitches during sleep.* Recurrent *boils,* itching skin. Dry, scaly, *unhealthy skin, with itching and burning:* offensive body odor. Worse from scratching and washing. Used for the chronic effects of illness. Likes fat. May be upset by eggs. Worse from washing, sleeping, rest, and warmth of bed. Better from dry, warm weather, lying on the right side.

Thuja

Thuja is a good remedy to give prior to and after *vaccination*: it counteracts ill effects from vaccinations. Sensation as if limbs were brittle and would break. Urethral and vaginal infections. Offensive smelling perspiration. *Headaches brought on by stress.* Persons who need this remedy are very *sensitive and maybe paranoid* that others are trying to manipulate them.

Final word about homeopathic home remedies

When choosing a remedy, it is not necessary that the subject demonstrates *all* symptoms as listed in the remedies above. You will be aiming to select the *best fit* for the 'symptom picture' of the person. Sometimes the same remedy will be the one used mostly when sickness occurs in an *individual.* As you see results your confidence in this method of healing will increase.

CHAPTER EIGHT

Bach Flower Remedies

The beauty of flowers to heal emotions

Flower essences have become popular throughout the world. Some countries produce their own unique flower essences, but the earliest known system of flower essences are Bach Flower Remedies named after Dr Edward Bach (1886 – 1936). This system and philosophy of vibrational medicine discovered by Dr Edward Bach treats the person not a disease. Dr Bach developed a system of medicine that considered the persons mental and emotional state which he believed contributed to their sickness and disease. Dr Bach, a medical practitioner dissatisfied with the medical system of his day, believed there should be a better way to treat the sick. Bach was a spiritual man and he was driven to find something better than the current medical system used. He fulfilled his destiny and life purpose when he began to wander the countryside of England searching to find gentle flower remedies that would heal the sick.[51]

Over a period of time Bach perfected his system of natural medicine and discovered 38 remedies derived from the flowers of wild plants, shrubs, or trees found in the English countryside. None of them were harmful or habit forming. They were not prescribed for the physical complaint that the person may present with but rather according to the patient's state of mind and emotions – to moods, fears, worry, anger, depression etc. After discovering his system of healing Bach seldom described diseases but viewed disease as resulting from a lack of harmony between soul, mind, and body. In the latter part of his life he always prescribed his Flower Remedies for the sick rather than drugs. Like homeopathy, these remedies have stood the test of time.

It is well known that a long-standing fear or worry can deplete an individual's vitality, causing the person to feel out of sorts, below par, or described as 'not him or herself'. Under these conditions the body loses its natural resistance to disease. When this happens, a person is open to infection and other forms of illness, whether it is a cold, rheumatism, headaches, digestive disturbances, or a more serious disease. It has been said that there are no diseases, only sick people, and when peace and harmony return to the mind, health and strength will return to the body. This provides a good picture of how the Bach Flower Remedies help to heal through the avenue of the mind and emotions.

Vlamis[20] reports how Bach worked to find the flower remedies. As his senses became highly refined he would experience the intense physical and mental symptoms of a disease. Then he would go into the fields and find the appropriate flower to match the symptoms he was experiencing. He would place a petal or flower in the palm of his hand, or on his tongue, and experience the effect of the plant on his mind and body.

Flower Remedies work through the subtle vibrational energy of plants, and for some people the subtle vibrational qualities of flowers seem rather esoteric, or even implausible. Yet, as people become spiritually sensitive and attuned to their natural environment this subtle realm of healing energy may become more of a daily reality as it was for Dr. Edward Bach.

Preparation and Manufacture of Remedies

The Bach Flower remedies are still prepared and manufactured by the Bach Flower Institute in England today, using Bach's original method.[21] The flowers are picked at a certain time on a sunny day and placed in a bowl of spring water. The flowers are left for a certain length of time. During this time the sun transmits the vibrational energy from the flowers to the water. This is the essential essence of the flower. The essence is then made into the concentrate that becomes 'stock'. A few drops of the stock are then used for making up individual prescriptions.

A Prescription

A prescription is generally made with three remedies (Bach recommended no more than three) yet other practitioners believe there can be up to five remedies in a prescription. I prefer to stay with three and follow up with a further three in a different prescription if required. The *Rescue Remedy* is a composite remedy with five different essences and this works really well when used for shock and stressful situations.

These Flower Remedies can be used for babies, children, animals, and plants. Taking a flower remedy alongside any other medicine is not a problem and can be taken with absolute safety. There is no danger of a harmful or conflicting result from prescribed medicine or a flower remedy when taken together.

How to make a remedy

To a small dropper bottle of water add three drops of each of the selected remedies from the stock remedy. Three drops of brandy may also be added to preserve the remedy if it is not being used immediately over the next few days.

How to take a remedy

Depending upon the need, a person may take the remedy once a day or several times a day. The remedy is taken until the fear/emotion/or problem has been overcome. It may be necessary to change the prescription as new fears, emotions, or other problems arise. If the wrong remedy is given it will not cause any harm but it will do no good either. Bach emphasised that the remedy must match the emotion and mental aspect and the person must be open to change for a total return to health. Often by just taking the correct remedy there *will* be a change in outlook, peace of mind, inner joy, and happiness as improvement takes place. The first remedy may be followed by a completely different remedy as new emotions surface.

List of the 39 Bach Flower remedies

1	Agrimony		2	Aspen	
3	Beech		4	Centaury	
5	Cerato		6	Cherry Plum	

7	Chestnut Bud	8	Chicory
9	Clematis	10	Crab Apple
11	Elm	12	Gentian
13	Gorse	14	Heather
15	Holly	16	Honeysuckle
17	Hornbeam	18	Impatiens
19	Larch	20	Mimulus
21	Mustard	22	Oak
23	Olive	24	Pine
25	Red Chestnut	26	Rock Rose
27	Rock Water	28	Scleranthus
29	Star of Bethlehem	30	Sweet Chestnut
31	Vervain	32	Vine
33	Walnut	34	Water Violet
35	White Chestnut	36	Wild Oat
37	Wild Rose	38	Willow
39	Rescue Remedy		

A Reference Key to Bach Flower Remedies

Following is a reference key that indicates major mental or emotional expressions that match each remedy.

Agrimony – for those not wanting to burden others with their troubles, so tend to put on a cheerful façade, to hide a worried mind.

Aspen – for vague fears and anxieties of unknown causes, a sense of foreboding, apprehension, or impending disaster.

Beech – desire perfection, easily find fault with people and things. Critical and intolerant, fail to find the good in others or a situation.

Centaury– Weakness of will: those who let themselves be exploited or imposed upon by others and who can allow themselves to become slaves. The individual who neglects their own needs and often becomes a doormat for others in life.

Cerato – Those who lack confidence in their own judgement, constantly seeking the advice of others, often becoming misguided.

Cherry Plum – Fear of mental collapse, of doing something desperate or known to be wrong- of the mind giving way. Uncontrolled temper.

Chestnut Bud – for those who fail to learn from experience, continually repeating the same patterns and mistakes.

Chicory – The over-possessive individual who is constantly seeking to put others right and demanding the attention of those close to them. Usually full of self-pity. Martyrs.

Clematis – The dreaming sort of person who pays little attention to what is going on in the environment. Lack of concentration, lack of interest in present circumstances.

Crab Apple – For those who feel unclean or ashamed of their ailments. A wonderful remedy for unsightly skin conditions. Self-condemnation.

Elm – For individuals who often overextend themselves and become overwhelmed with feelings of inadequacy and responsibility.

Gentian – Individuals with feelings of discouragement, self-doubt and depression.

Gorse – for individuals with feelings of despair, hopelessness, and utter despondency.

Heather – for those talkative individuals who constantly seek the companionship of anyone who will listen to their troubles. They are self-absorbed, generally poor listeners, and don't like being alone.

Holly – For individuals who are jealous, envious, revengeful, and suspicious. For those who hate others. All negative feelings that indicate a need for love.

Honeysuckle – For individuals with nostalgia and who constantly dwell in the past. Homesickness.

Hornbeam – For individuals who feel too exhausted to deal with their daily duties, although they usually succeed in fulfilling their task. 'Monday morning' feeling.

Impatiens – Impatience, irritability, mental tension.

Larch - Despondency due to lack of self-confidence, expectation of failure so the individual fails to make the attempt and consequently feels inferior.

Mimulus – Fear of known things, for example, fear of heights, spiders, and darkness.

Mustard – Dark depression which descends upon the individual for no known cause or reason and can lift just as suddenly.

Oak – Despair but never giving up, the individual is brave and struggles on despite despondency, a plodder.

Olive – Exhaustion and utter weariness. Tiredness, both mental and physical. The individual suffers under adverse conditions for a long time.

Pine – For the individual who has feelings of guilt and considers that they should do better. They often blame themselves for the mistakes of others.

Red Chestnut – The individual has an excessive fear or anxiety for others, such as an over-protective mother.

Rock Rose – An individual in extreme terror, panic, hysteria, or very frightened and has nightmares.

Rock Water – For individuals who martyr themselves in their pursuit of an ideal, rigid minded and inflexible. Self-denial is a keyword.

Scleranthus – Uncertainty and indecision, for individuals who are unable to decide between two choices, first one seeming right then the other.

Star of Bethlehem – For all kinds of shock, for the after effects of trauma, whether emotional or physical. For example, for grief, loss, or after an accident.

Sweet Chestnut – For the despair of individuals who feel they have reached the limits of endurance, but not suicidal. For dark despair, where the anguish seems to be unbearable.

Vervain – The over-enthusiastic individual, over-effort, straining, fanatical and highly-strung, tense, incensed by injustices. Individuals who have very strong opinions.

Vine – Climber, dominating and inflexible, ruthless and crave power. Autocratic, dictatorial, ruthless.

Walnut – This remedy gives protection to the individual from outside influences. The over sensitive individual. This remedy acts as a link-breaker for times of transition and change in life e.g., teething, puberty, marriage, separation, menopause, changing jobs, shifting house etc.

Water Violet – Proud, aloof, 'superior' condescending individuals who do not interfere in the affairs of others.

White Chestnut – Individuals with persistent, unwanted thoughts, and mental pre-occupation with some worry or episode.

Wild Oat – Dissatisfaction with not having found one's goal in life, but not really knowing what it is.

Wild Rose – for individuals who are apathetic and have resigned themselves to their circumstances, making little effort to improve things or to find joy in life.

Willow – Resentment and bitterness towards others, takers not givers.

Rescue Remedy – a composite of Cherry Plum, Clematis, Impatiens, Rock Rose and Star of Bethlehem. This is an all-purpose remedy for shock, terror, emotional upsets, stage fright, exams, dental work, surgery or any trauma whether minor or serious. It is strongly advised that everyone have this remedy on hand for rescue situations (self or someone else) to be given after any kind of trauma. It is a pre-eminent *First Aid* remedy.

Another approach to view Dr Bach's 38 remedies is within seven major emotional and psychological categories: fear, uncertainty, insufficient interest in present conditions, loneliness, oversensitivity, despondency or despair, and over-care for the welfare of others.

Fear

- Rock Rose   extreme terror
- Mimulus   fear of known
- Aspen   fear of unknown
- Cherry Plum   fear of losing control
- Red Chestnut   excessive fear for others

Uncertainty

- Cerato   doubt of one's ability
- Sclerathus   indecision
- Gentian   doubt and depression
- Gorse   hopelessness and despair
- Hornbeam   wariness
- Wild Oat   dissatisfaction

Insufficient Interest in Present Conditions

- Clematis   indifference
- Honeysuckle   dwelling in the past

- Wild Rose   apathy
- Olive   exhaustion
- White Chestnut   unwanted thoughts
- Mustard   black depression
- Chestnut Bud   failure to learn from experience

Loneliness

- Water Violet   aloof
- Impatiens   impatience
- Heather   self-centred

Oversensitivity

- Agrimony   mental torture
- Centaury   weak willed
- Walnut   link breaker
- Holly   anger

Despondency Or Despair

- Larch   lack of confidence
- Pine   guilt
- Elm   over-striving for perfection
- Sweet Chestnut   anguish
- Star of Bethlehem   shock
- Willow   bitterness
- Crab Apple   cleansing

Overcare For The Welfare Of Others

- Chicory   possessive
- Vervain   over enthusiastic
- Vine   dominating
- Beech   intolerance
- RockWater   rigidity

Stock Bottles

A full set of 39 stock remedies can be purchased from the *Dr Bach Centre*, England.[52] This set of remedies normally come in 10ml bottles and will keep indefinitely. They need to be kept stored in a cool place.

Preparation of a remedy from stock

Decide which remedy or remedies the individual requires. If two or more, combine them in the same bottle. Choose no more than five remedies at a time for any one bottle to ensure the chosen preparation does its best work.

Into a bottle (up to 30ml) add 2 drops from each of the stock bottles chosen.

Add a teaspoonful of Brandy to act as a preservative – this is optional and not necessary if the remedy is being used immediately and not kept for any length of time. Fill the bottle with clean pure water. Store bottle in a cool place especially in a warm climate.

Daily dosage

Three drops three times a day. The Bach Remedies are never harmful and taking extra does not increase their effectiveness. Children are given the same dose as adults. In severe cases, such as shock or fever, the remedy may be given frequently (every 5 minutes) until the person feels better.

Rescue Remedy

One of the most valuable remedies is Rescue Remedy. If you choose to have only one remedy, then this is the one to always have handy. You will be able to use this remedy for all manner of problems. You may be able to purchase a bottle from your local pharmacy, chemist, health food shop or naturopath.

The composite Rescue Remedy is made up of the following five Bach Flower Remedies:

o   Impatiens – for the impatience, irritability, and agitation often accompanying stress. It helps muscle tension and pain.
o   Clematis – for unconsciousness, spaciness, faintness, and out-of-the-body sensations, which often accompany accidents and trauma (physical or emotional).

o   Rock Rose – for terror, panic, hysteria, great fear.
o   Cherry Plum – for fear of losing mental or physical control.
o   Star of Bethlehem – for trauma, both mental and physical.

Rescue remedy is excellent to stabilise people in a state of shock, (physical or emotional). It is useful during stressful situations, or any emotional crisis at all. It is an excellent *First Aid* remedy for children or adults. Use this remedy in every-day life: before and after the dentist, before and after a stressful meeting, before an exam, after receiving bad news, after an accident, when feeling faint or fearful, the list goes on and on and in fact it can be useful for any reason whatsoever. When an individual is in great distress – give every five minutes until relief is obtained, then administer less frequently until the person is stable again. However, only take when necessary to gain full effect.

Rescue Remedy can be purchased as a stock remedy and can be used direct from the stock bottle. If you purchase a stock bottle it will generally last a long time. Further bottles can be made from the stock bottle for everyday use by adding 5 drops of stock remedy to a 30ml bottle of pure water and adding a few drops of brandy to preserve it (if necessary). Keep a bottle in the kitchen, one in the car, and another in your handbag or briefcase.

Animals, birds (particularly ones the cat catches), and plants, can be treated successfully with Rescue Remedy too!

Make a bottle of Rescue Remedy from Stock Bottles:

If you have stock bottles of impatiens, clematis, rock rose, cherry plum and star of Bethlehem, then you can make your own bottle of Rescue Remedy from your own stock.

Add 2 drops from each of the stock bottles (5 remedies listed above) to 30ml water with a few drops of brandy as a preservative (if necessary).

How to use the Rescue Remedy

Rescue Remedy is generally purchased in a dropper bottle, so you can squirt 2 – 4 drops directly into the mouth or add 4 drops of Rescue Remedy to a glass of water. Sip frequently at first, then lengthen the time to 15 minutes, then 30 minutes, and longer intervals as improvement begins.

If the person is unconscious, rub Rescue Remedy on lips, gums, behind the ears, and on the wrists, it can be used direct from the bottle in this way.

To apply to external injuries and stings: use 6 drops of Rescue Remedy to half a cupful of water and bathe the injury with it or apply a compress soaked in the water.

Preparing your own flower essences

You may like to experiment and prepare your own flower Essences using the sunshine method.

The Sunshine Method Requires:

A clear glass bowl.

Uncontaminated spring or clean stream water is ideal.

Clean bottles and labels.

Clean jug or a funnel to pour water from the bowl into bottles.

Brandy as a preservative.

The procedure should be carried out on a clear, sunny day - preferably late spring or early summer when the sun is at its highest point. Morning is the best time of day because this is the time to harness energy from the rising sun which will energise the essence.

Choose an area where the selected flowers are growing in abundance and create your own ritual for attuning yourself to nature.

Fill the glass bowl with water.

Pick blossoms and float them immediately on the surface of the water in the bowl. It is recommended that you handle the flowers with a leaf or stem from the plant to avoid touching the blossoms or the water. Continue adding blossoms to the water until the surface is fully covered, and each blossom is touching the water.

Place the bowl carefully where it will not be disturbed and let it remain fully exposed to the sunshine. After about three hours – less if the blossoms begin fading, carefully remove the flowers from the bowl, again using plant parts so that you are not touching the water.

The bottles are half-filled with the sun-potentized flower essence water and an equal amount of brandy is then added to act as a natural preservative. This forms the *Mother Essence*. Shake well.

Stock Essence is prepared by adding two drops of the *Mother Essence* to a

30 ml (or one ounce) bottle filled with a mixture of half brandy (optional) and half clean uncontaminated water. Shake well.

Individual dosage bottles are prepared by adding two drops of stock essence into a 30 ml bottle of water with a few drops of brandy preservative (amount will vary according to the length of time the bottle will be stored). Shake well.

With each dilution, tapping or shaking the bottle against your hand can help release the energy of the essence.

It is important to remember that flower essence preparation is more than formulae and mechanical procedures. The essential aspect is an inter-relationship of consciousness between human, plant, and natural elemental energies (see *Wellness Model Fig. 1*). Attunement, purity of mind, and love creates the energy in this process that forms the foundation of flower essence preparation.

A word about metaphysics

Metaphysics is a step beyond homeopathy and Bach Flower Remedies. In metaphysics matter disappears and a higher state of Mind (or 'S') takes over to effectively heal.

Once you begin to tune into your environment you will recognise trees, plants, and flowers *all* have vibrational healing energies and all you need to do is to enter their environment to receive healing energy. Try hugging a tree, stand with your back against a tree, or breathe in the scent of a rose. Sit and let your eyes absorb the vibration from bright yellow flowers (or any other flower), stand in bare feet on sand, or earth, or green grass. Notice how your mind and emotions are affected and problems disappear. Let yourself just be in the moment and you will begin to feel stress disappear, you will begin to feel uplifted, and energised! This is all part of a wellness model you can enter to heal and sustain health.

> *"Every single person has a life to live, a work to do, a*
> *glorious personality, a wonderful individuality"*
> Dr Edward Bach

CHAPTER NINE

Herbal Remedies for Home Help

Herbs have been said to be 'weeds with a purpose' – all herbs are not exactly weeds but there are certainly many nutritious weeds growing everywhere. Most herbs will grow like weeds: we will discuss some of the common home herbs that are nutritional, medicinal, cosmetic, and that also deter troublesome insects from the environment when used in various ways.

If you intend to use herbal remedies in conjunction with, or as an alternative to, medical drugs then it is advisable to first discuss the matter with your doctor. This risk is increased when herbal remedies are taken in combination with prescription, pharmaceutical or any other drug. For example, if you are taking pharmaceutical drugs to lower blood pressure, and at the same time take an herbal supplement with the same affect, there is a risk of blood pressure dropping dangerously low. Keep in mind that herbal remedies can cause adverse reactions similar to conventional drugs. Herbal remedies tend to work more on physical symptoms of disease, rather than the subtle vibrational level that Homeopathic and Bach Flower Remedies work best on. Nevertheless, *living* herbs do have a vital, vibrational energy too and will treat the whole person when taken in their natural unadulterated state.

History of herbs

The oldest known herbal book, *Herbal and Medical Experiment Poisons*, was the work of an ancient Chinese emperor Shen Nung believed to have lived 5000 years ago. He is called the Father of Chinese Medicine and noted for tasting 365 herbs and dying of a toxic overdose.

Out of Egypt came papyrus scrolls called *The Papyrus Ebers*, an ancient text written in 1500 BC that contains references to more than 700 herbal remedies. Many remedies mentioned were majoram, mint. basil, parsley, anise, dill, and garlic, to name a few we use today to sustain health.

Romans were influenced by Greek knowledge of herbs, and Roman soldiers carried herbs on the march, in particular thyme as it was believed to prevent food poisoning by eating it before and after a meal.

The renaissance saw herbal cultivation spread beyond the gardens of royalty and religious orders, and into gardens and kitchens of commoners. All indigenous peoples have had their own herbal wisdom and carried it over the centuries - the Celtic English, European, Indian, America Indian, Maori of Pacifica and New Zealand. For many people their traditional way of living - growing, harvesting, and using herbs continues.

Doctrine of signatures

It is said that there is a key to the use of every herb. Called the 'doctrine of signatures' whereby nature has left a mark upon the plant (within the flower, leaf, or root) so that humans can recognize and understand how to use the plant by matching what it looks like with a specific part of the human body. This herbal lore stems from the belief that everything is part of the one universal energy system (Spirit 'S') and that nature has consciousness and meaning. If we read these signs and understand the laws of nature, we will know among other things, how to cure ourselves.[53]

Many herbal medicines can be grown in the home garden, in pots, on a patio, or inside. People often start growing a few herbs that can be used in cooking, in salads, and in teas, then develop a wider interest in medicinal herbs. Herbs freshly picked raw are best because they are nutritionally superior to dried or processed herbs. Herbs can be your medicine when sick or unwell and they will sustain you when you are well. Fresh from their natural state herbs are a super vitamin and mineral supplement in an easily digestible balanced form.

Always keep in mind that unlike conventional medicines natural herbal remedies take time to show their full effect. Herbal medicines work more gradually as they feed the physical body the substances it needs as they do their healing work.

Herbal remedies described here are ones that can be easily grown at home, either in the country or city. By growing a few herbs, you will have instant vibrant living remedies at your disposal to sustain health and treat sickness if it arises.

There are several different ways to use herbs at home – raw, infusions, decoctions, tinctures, poultices, or creams. If you don't grow herbs yourself they can be purchased in various forms from retail outlets – dried in capsules, tablets, liquid mixtures, and as tinctures. Be aware that *sometimes processed herbal remedies will have only one part extracted from the plant so may have a different effect than consuming a plant in its natural living state.* Herbs concentrated and processed into pills or potions may have side effects for some people too. Sometimes it is preferable to consult an Herbalist, or a Naturopath trained in prescribing herbs for advice on the correct form of remedy to take. Often a professional will mix an individual prescription for a client. It is wise if taking pharmaceutical drugs, to consult your medical practitioner before taking processed herbal remedies in case there is any incompatibility with medicines you are taking. For example the herb St Johns wort and the herb Gingko do not work well with anti-depressants drugs.

Raw Herbal remedy

As the name suggests raw herbal medicine is taken in its most natural form and its most vital and energised state. Parsley is one of the best raw remedies and it is easy to grow in a container on the patio or in the garden. A sprig of parsley freshly picked and eaten every day provides a natural balanced and energizing vitamin and mineral supplement. Other common raw herbal remedies are thyme, sage, basil, marjoram, garlic, and chives to name a few that are easy to grow.

Concentrated juice

Juice from raw herbs is a concentrate. Chop or crush a small amount of the herbs to squeeze out the juice (don't use a blender). Add water to the juice concentrate and drink it immediately. Do not store juice for more than a day extracted this way. Always make it fresh.

Herbal Infusions.

Herbal infusions are the most popular way to take herbs on a regular basis. Infusions are quick to make and easy to administer. Infusions are mostly tea-like beverages that are made by adding boiled water to fresh or dried herbs. Leaves, seeds, and fruits of a plant can be used for an infusion. To make an infusion the common method is steeping by pouring boiling water over the herbs in a cup, porcelain jug, or teapot. Typical ratios are about half to one ounce of herbs to one pint (600mls) of boiling water. Leave for five to ten minutes to infuse (steep). Strain into a cup and either sip or drink the infusion when cool.

Some examples of herbs used for teas are stinging nettle, oat straw, red clover, raspberry leaf, rosemary, parsley, sage, thyme, and comfrey (young comfrey leaves are best). Black tea, red-bush (rooibush) tea, and green tea are infusions that many people drink every day and are all good sources of antioxidants.

"Medicinal" infusions are usually a more concentrated and stronger tea – for example, a strong black tea (traditional) can be taken to relieve a tension headache. Both black and green teas are excellent antioxidants and help to remove toxic material from the body cells. A sweetener such as honey, or a slice of lemon, may be added if desired.

Cold extracts are made using cold instead of boiling water. The advantage is that cold, unlike hot water, allows some of the more volatile ingredients in herbs to be preserved and not wasted in the extraction process. To prepare cold extracts, double the amount of herbal material and let it sit in cold water for twelve hours and then strain the mixture before drinking it.

Herbal Poultice

Herbal poultices are remedies applied to the skin and used for old injuries, inflammation, or to draw something to a head beneath the skin and encourage it to burst out through the skin such as a boil, infection, thistle, or splinter of wood.

To make a poultice the required herbs are first chopped or ground into small pieces. These are then either applied directly to the affected area, or applied on a cotton cloth to the area, and covered with a hot, moist bandage. This can then be covered with a piece of plastic, to retain heat and moisture, and bandaged with a dry bandage to keep the poultice in place. Every four hours apply a fresh poultice. Oat straw, oats, comfrey, thyme, and sage, all make excellent poultices for skin infections and healing rough skin. Crushed broccoli is useful as a poultice for skin cancer.

Herbal Tincture

Herbal tinctures are strong herbal medicines in a concentrated liquid form. The herbal goodness is extracted with alcohol. Tinctures are best used externally for cuts and bruises to cleanse and heal them. Arnica and calendula are two very good tinctures that can be used for minor bruises and injuries – particularly handy for childhood scrapes and bruises. A strong tincture will sometimes sting so for children's open cuts and bruises dilute the tincture with water or use an oil or ointment instead.

To make a tincture at home:

- Pack the herbs into a small jar
- Cover with alcohol. Brandy or vodka can be used for the alcohol base.
- Cover the jar and leave for three weeks.
- Strain off the herbs.
- Use the tincture when required.
- This tincture keeps well.

Herbal Decoction

Herbal decoctions are liquid preparations made by boiling a medicinal plant with water to extract the medicinal properties. The end product, the decoction, is a concentration of the mixture that has been reduced to half the original amount. The slowly boiling of the mixture will extract the medicinal ingredients and reduce it to half the original quantity. Typically, specific parts of a plant like berries, roots, or bark are used in this process.

When preparing your herbal remedies always use a non-metallic or enamel pot.

Usual proportions are 5 parts of the plant to 100 parts of water and for a small quantity 1/2 ounce of herbs with one cup of water. Bring the mixture to boil, then turn down to boil slowly until it is half the original quantity. Keep the lid on the pot and be patient because this may take up to two hours or longer to prepare. It is important to keep the lid on because it retains the essence of the herb in the pot and nothing is lost.

Oat straw and dandelion root are both excellent decoctions to internally cleanse the body.

Herbal Syrup

Herbal syrups are useful for children and persons who are unable to swallow a bitter herbal remedy. A syrup can be made in the same way as a decoction or a raw remedy. To the prepared decoction add raw sugar or honey until it dissolves and overcomes the bitter taste.

An excellent raw syrup for a sore throat is to cut up an onion (or garlic). Cover the onion with either raw sugar or honey and leave for one hour. During this time the medicinal qualities will be drawn from the onion (or garlic) into the sugar (or honey) and this mixture can be taken by the teaspoonful to soothe and heal a sore throat.

Herbal Powder

An herbal powder can be made from grinding dried herbs. First you will need to dry the herb in a warm, airy space, and then store in an airtight jar. Either grind the herbs as soon as they are dry and store in an airtight container, or, grind up dried herbs just before use. The powder can then be taken with water, milk, or added to soup, or other recipes. Most culinary herbs sold in retail outlets are dried and ground ready for use.

Herbal Ointment

Herbal ointments can be prepared by adding olive oil to a previously prepared decoction and then simmered over a low heat until the water has evaporated. Beeswax may be added to improve the consistency of the ointment. Mix well.

Another ointment can be made with vaseline or glycerine as the base. Although vaseline is inorganic it has the advantage that an ointment can be made quickly. The vaseline acts as a carrier only and will not be absorbed through the skin. Melt the vaseline over a low heat and add freshly picked and chopped herbs. Simmer gently for ten minutes, strain through gauze and squeeze out all the liquid. Store in jars.

Herbal Oil

To make an herbal oil place herbs in a clear glass jar and cover with an appropriate oil such as olive, coconut, almond or sunflower oil. Leave outside in the sunshine or on a windowsill exposed to the sun for two weeks. Shake every day. After two weeks strain and use the oil. To make the oil stronger, keep adding fresh herbs to the oil every day for the first week. After two or three weeks, strain the oil and it is ready for use.

Lavender plus almond oil makes a nice massage oil. Lavender and coconut oil is good for sunburn. A mixture of wild plantain and coconut oil repels mosquitos and other insects when applied to the skin, and heals their bites too. Plantain makes a good all-round healing oil or ointment for cuts and sores on the skin.

Twelve of the best and most versatile herbs for home use:

Aloe Vera

Every household should have an Aloe Vera plant growing either in the garden or in a pot somewhere. It is easy to grow, and it is a very versatile herb. Aloe Vera requires minimal care except for a little water and protection from frosts in winter and it will reproduce regularly. You can detach the small plants as they sprout from the base of the mother plant and give them away to friends and neighbours.

Aloe Vera is one of the best remedies for burns, particularly kitchen burns, either dry burns, or scalding water burns. It is good for sunburn as well. Aloe Vera is excellent for any inflammation, skin rashes, and skin burning from an allergy, insect bite, sting, hemorrhoids, herpes virus (cold sores and genital herpes). Chronic leg ulcers, cuts and scratches that have become inflamed, will all benefit from a dressing of Aloe Vera gel. Other uses of Aloe Vera include skin beauty, helps to prevent wrinkles, and assists hair growth. It can be a soothing treatment for arthritis and rheumatism.

Internal uses include stimulating enzymes in the digestive system, stimulating the flow of bile, as a general tonic, and to heal stomach ulcers. Aloe Vera taken internally needs to be diluted 1:10.

Application for external use:

- With any herbal remedy, give thanks, remove and use only as much as is required.
- Take an older leaf off the plant. It is possible to break a large leaf in half and it will naturally seal itself at the break.
- Peel the outside layer of thick green skin from the leaf and expose the gelatinous substance inside.
- Scrape the gel off the leaf.
- Apply the gel directly to the area to be treated.
- Continue to apply gel - it will dry and form a skin over the treated area.

For hair care and baldness, massage the gel into hair roots.
To make a face pack

- Half a teaspoonful of Aloe Vera gel
- 1 teaspoonful of rolled oats
- Juice of half a lemon
- Mix together rolled oats with the lemon juice
- Add Aloe Vera gel and mix
- Add a little milk to make a smooth paste.
- Apply to the face and leave 30 minutes.
- Wash off.

Basil

Basil is an easy to grow herb and can be used for headache, nausea, and rheumatism Basil can be made into an infusion, as well as being useful in many culinary dishes.

Use the tops and leaves of basil on vegetables, in salads, soups, and dressings.

It is tasty eaten when eaten with egg, tomato and onion dishes.

Calendula

Calendula officinalis or the beautiful English marigold, grows easily, reproduces well, and will provide an endless supply of sunshine yellow and orange flowers. It is an excellent anti-inflammatory herb and is best known for its action on the skin.

Use for inflammation, cuts, bruises, bleeding, slow healing wounds, ulcers, for minor burns and scalds.

Calendula can be used as an infusion, tincture, ointment, poultice, or compress.

Coriander

Coriander stimulates the appetite and is an aid to digestion. It helps reduce blood sugar levels and strengthens the heart. It is useful to relieve rheumatism and arthritis. An eyewash from coriander tea has a mild antibacterial action.

Coriander has multiple uses in the kitchen; fresh young leaves for salads, soups and curries. Dried seeds can be used in curries, cakes, baked or stewed apples.

Dill

Dill is one of the best remedies for mothers, babies and children. Dill is useful to increase mothers milk flow when breast feeding a baby. A tea made with dill seeds makes a soothing remedy for babies who suffer from 'wind', gas and digestive problems. This herb is an excellent digestive aid and can be used for hiccups. Chewing seeds removes bad breath. Other uses of dill are for ulcers, swellings, pains, and urinary infections. This herb reduces blood pressure and helps reduce weight.

Fresh dill leaves make an excellent tea or use up to one teaspoonful of seeds to a cup of boiling water instead. Dill is a useful herb in the kitchen for salads as well as cooking fish, steak, and lamb chops. Use seeds when making pickles.

Garlic

Garlic is one of the best-known natural antibiotics and is extremely effective in destroying pathogenic bacteria so it can be used in cases of infection, either internally or externally.

For sore throats, coughs, and influenza consider garlic as a remedy. Castleman[23] suggests one medium sized clove is equivalent to 1000,000 units of penicillin. Garlic is also useful to expel intestinal worms and for fungal infections such as candida.

- Chop up or crush several garlic cloves.
- Add honey to cover, stir well and leave for one hour.
- Take by the teaspoonful for all manner of complaints.

Add one or more cloves of crushed garlic to a bowl of cooked porridge. Taken on a daily basis during winter months garlic will sustain well-being and help prevent ailments such as coughs and influenza.

An antidote to garlic odour on the breath is to chew parsley, or drink milk.

Unfortunately, some people are sensitive to garlic, if this is the case the next best option is to use onion instead, which is milder yet has similar effects to garlic.

Lavender

There are many varieties of Lavender, some are easier to grow than others, and some produce more oil than others, but all lavenders have a special place in many gardens and are an extremely useful herb to grow.

Lavender is a plant with many healing properties particularly for winter ailments, infectious diseases, and any bacterial induced sickness, for migraines, epilepsy and insomnia.

Use fresh lavender flowers to make an oil to rub onto the chest for chest complaints and to massage into rheumatic and arthritic joints to relieve pain. A Lavender tea taken on an empty stomach will destroy worms in the intestines. Lavender flowers in little muslin bags can be placed in drawers and cupboards to deter insects and leave a sweet smell. Keep lavender in the kitchen to deter flies. Small bags of lavender, leaves and flowers, can be placed inside a pillowcase to induce sleep. Take a hot relaxing bath by adding sprigs of lavender to the water.

Parsley

Parsley is one of the most commonly used herbs for culinary dishes and fresh salads. As mentioned previously, chewing a sprig every day is a superb vitamin and mineral supplement. It is an excellent blood purifier and beneficial for cleansing the kidneys. It improves the strength of the heart muscle and is a valuable herb for anyone suffering from arthritis and rheumatism. Externally it can eliminate freckles from the skin, relieve the itch of hives, and have a beneficial effect on some skin cancers. Eat a few leaves raw every day, add to salads and soups, take as a tea, or use as a compress on the skin.

Peppermint

Peppermint relieves all forms of fever, flatulence, nausea, vomiting, diarrhoea, anxiety, stress, tired muscles, stiff and aching joints. It is useful as a tonic during pregnancy and will alleviate nausea and discomforts associated with pregnancy. Peppermint leaves can be used direct from the garden and added to salads. For a refreshing drink add a few leaves to a cup of boiling water. As a cool drink fresh peppermint leaves can be added to cold water.

As a nerve tonic peppermint tea is excellent, especially for headaches, migraine, insomnia, stress and anxiety. Also, peppermint tea will relieve coughs and colds, fever, asthma, bronchitis, and other chest infections. Make your own peppermint oil or purchase a concentrated essential oil of peppermint from retail outlets to have on hand for first aid use in the home. Essential oil will be much stronger than any home-made oil and can be administered for many. Complaints, care must be taken with internal administration of any concentrated *essential oil* because in large doses they can be toxic. It can be applied to the body, or, in the case of colds and chest complaints – make an inhalation. Only one or two drops of essential peppermint oil in an inhalation is sufficient.

Peppermint oil has been found useful in treating herpes simplex and toothache. Take care when applying to the tooth or skin – use an ear bud and only a little oil directly on the spot required.

There is a whole range of mint plants available that are useful for teas too. Common garden mint can be used in salads, to add flavor when cooking potatoes, and for making a mint sauce (with vinegar) as a dressing for roast lamb.

Rosemary

Like Lavender, there are many different kinds of rosemary, they all have similar qualities and are relatively easy to grow. Once established they will grow for years and they can be grown very effectively from cuttings. The flowers and leaves of the rosemary plant have a wide range of uses.

Nervous and tension headaches, poor memory, failing vision, digestive disturbances, colic in babies, respiratory problems. Useful for sore throats and hay fever. Rosemary improves circulation, raises blood pressure, and strengthens a weak heart muscle. It improves supply of mother's milk and assists menstruation. It is useful to get rid of nits and head lice. Excellent for alleviating aches and pains of muscles and joints such as arthritis, rheumatism, and sports injuries.

For most conditions and as a tonic - make a tea with a sprig of rosemary and take three cups throughout the day. A teaspoonful of weak tea given to infants will relieve colic in most cases. Sore eyes can be bathed in a strong rosemary tea solution.

Mixture for a hair conditioner and to eradicate nits and lice:

- One part of Olive Oil.
- One part of Apple Cider Vinegar.
- Add fresh rosemary leaves and flowers (if no flowers available then leaves alone will do). If no fresh rosemary is available, then 2 drops of essential oil of rosemary can be used.
- Shake well.
- Leave 24 hours.
- Shake again and it is ready for use.
- Rub into scalp.

Sage

Sage is well known as an herb to improve memory and restore the voice. For a sore throat and loss of voice (useful for singers who overuse their voice), chop fresh sage finely, add the juice of a lemon and honey to taste. Drinking sage tea is a good tonic for improving memory. Fresh or dried sage leaves can be used in salads, soups, and stews.

Pimples and acne

- Chop up fresh sage leaves.
- Cover with apple cider vinegar.
- Bring to boil.

- Simmer with the lid on for ten minutes.
- Strain and cool.
- Dab this mixture onto the pimples and acne frequently.
- Also drink sage tea.

Thyme

There are many species of thyme and all have therapeutic properties. The best-known use for thyme is as an antiseptic, internal or external. Therefore, it is useful as a tea for sore throats, coughs, colds, chest infections, and digestive upsets. Use externally on the skin for any infection, scabies, athletes foot, and eczema. It can be used as a mouthwash to freshen the mouth too. As a digestive aid it can be used fresh in salads, or fresh and dried in cooking. Thyme and sage are two herbs traditionally used by some cultures in stuffing for meat dishes and other recipes in the kitchen.

Ginger and Turmeric

These two herbs come from the same family and are widely used in cooking throughout the world. Although not commonly grown in New Zealand home gardens they are, however, available from retail stores. Because they are extremely useful I have included them here in the hope that you may experiment in growing your own ginger and turmeric.

Both herbs have antioxidant and anti-inflammatory properties. They are currently popular as anti-cancer herbs. Ginger is excellent to treat nausea from any cause and will provide relief for an upset stomach. Ginger works well with the immune system to prevent disease and is capable of destroying streptococcal and staphylococcal infections. It is also useful for treating fungal infections. Tumeric is a valuable antioxidant and anti-inflammatory herb because of its curcumin content. Its usefulness includes a wide range of health benefits for muscles, joints, cardiovascular and digestive systems. The secret for ultimate absorption of turmeric is to include black pepper when using it. Ginger and turmeric can be used as a tea and in cooking or the powdered herb can be sprinkled on food.

The above herbal remedies are just a few of the many available from my cultural roots that I know will sustain wellness. You may come from a completely different culture, maybe Maori, Pacific Islander, Indian, Malaysian, Chinese, Greek, Italian, or another - discover the benefits of the herbs your culture has traditionally used. Get to know and use a few herbs well and you will find they will serve you throughout life. Grow herbs in your garden, or in pots on the patio, and you will always have something to enrich the flavour of your food, as well as having medicines available for immediate use.

Love and look after your herbs and they will look after you.

CHAPTER TEN

Aromatherapy

Smell (aroma) affects our lives and emotions in ways that scientists are only now beginning to explore. Aromatherapy has been used for centuries by many civilisations throughout the world. Ancient cultures instinctively looked to nature for cures of their physical, emotional, and spiritual ailments and many fragrant flowers, herbs, and oils were used as cures.

History of Aromatherapy

One of the earliest records of aromatherapy was found in Egyptian hieroglyphics dated around 3000BC. It showed that ancient Egyptian priests and priestesses used aromatic oils in their rituals and for healing.

There are various references in the *Holy Bible* to the use of essential oils, for example, God directed Moses to make holy anointing oil from myrrh, sweet cinnamon, calamus, cassia, and olive oil. Knowing their constituents nowadays we understand that this would have been a powerful anti-viral and antibiotic oil, the use of which gave protection and treatment to all those to whom it was administered.

The Roman and the Greek civilisations used essential oils in their public baths and employed massage and aromatic oils to maintain good health.

During the 'Black Death' plague in England smelly oils were used extensively - mainly for fumigation. Aromatic woods such as pine were lit in the streets. Essential oils such as peppermint and rosemary were an integral part of the herbalist's medicine box at that time mainly due to their antiseptic properties. The belief that oils could destroy the plague from the air was correct. As a child during an influenza epidemic I recall my mother walking around the house with a hand shovel of red hot coals to which a rather repugnant oil had been added to fumigate the house. This produced a smelly smoke that filtered through the air, and no doubt played a part in protecting our rather large family from the epidemic.

In 1937 the term "Aromatherapie" was first used by a French chemist Rene Maurice Gattefosse to describe the therapeutic action of aromatic plant essences. While making fragrance's one day in his laboratory, he burnt his arm very badly and thrust it into the nearest cold liquid which happened to be a tub of lavender oil. He was surprised to find that the pain lessened considerably and did not develop into a red, hot, inflamed area with blisters. His burn healed very quickly and left no scar at all. From that day forward, he devoted his life to discovering and researching the healing properties of aromatic or essential oils.

Around the same time as Gattefosse was doing his research during World War II, Dr Jean Valnet discovered the regenerative and antiseptic qualities of essential oils while treating soldiers war injuries. Although penicillin began to be used during this period he discarded penicillin in favour of essential oils. He wrote *The Practice of Aromatherapy* in 1980[24] which has become a very popular book about the use of essential oils.

One of Dr Valnet's students, Marguerite Maury, a biochemist who lived in France, began to use essential oils with massage and she is credited with introducing aromatherapy to England. Today aromatherapy is used extensively all over the world and in all cultures and is considered a professional healing modality.

How does aromatherapy work?

Essential oils are thought to affect the body in two ways. The first and most obvious is through the sense of smell during breathing. On the inward breath anything in the air travels through the nose and reaches the brain first through the cribiform plate of the ethmoid bone which is a bony structure with little holes to allow olfactory nerves to pass to the nose. Behind the cribiform plate is the olfactory bulb at the base of the cranial cavity and it is from here that fibers enter the frontal lobe of the brain and also the limbic system through the rhinoencehalon part of the brain.

The air continues to move through the nasal passages into the lungs and from the lungs this oxygenated air enters the blood stream and flows to every part of the body. The ability to perceive odour is so connected to our well-being that people who have lost their sense of smell often suffer from a high incidence of depression and anxiety.

How scent is perceived and processed in the brain is a complicated physical and sensory process, which is not yet fully understood. We are aware however, of all the body senses smell has the most direct and most instant connection to the mind and emotions. All fragrances, natural or synthetic, are able to breach the blood brain barrier (the protective membrane that surrounds the brain) and gain direct access to the limbic system, considered the emotional switchboard of the brain.

Aromatherapy oils can also enter the blood stream through the skin when applied directly to it especially when used in massage oils. Aromatherapy no doubt works on the mind and body at the same time. In therapeutic use there are about 150 essential oils distilled from plants, flowers, trees, bark, nuts, grasses, and seeds. Each has a distinctive chemical make-up and a unique therapeutic, psychological, and physiological effect. Some are antiseptic, others are antiviral, anti-inflammatory, pain relieving, antidepressant, or expectorant. They can be used within the body, to stimulate energy, relax the nervous system, improve digestion, and eliminate excess water.

Extraction of essential oils

For effective use in healing it is vital that only a "pure" essential oil is used. This oil is the natural plant essence which has been extracted by either steam distillation, solvent extraction, expression, maceration or enfleurage. There is no point buying a product that is called a fragrance (rather than an essential oil) no matter how charming its aroma, because it is a reconstituted product or a chemical copy of the natural essence. These simply do not work in the same manner as naturally extracted essential oils because they do not have the same therapeutic value. Sometimes it is difficult to tell the difference, but surprisingly essential oils *do not* feel oily when extracted from a plant, so the feel test is a good guide as to whether the oil is truly a natural essential oil or not. Essential oils are concentrated so it takes a lot of herbs to make a small amount of essential oil.

Steam distillation

Plants are heated by steam in equipment for distilling. The essential oil is released by heat and evaporates into steam. It is then carried along a pipe that passes through cold water which cools the steam and is returned back to its liquid form. When the liquid comes out of the distiller the essential oil floats on the surface of the water and can then be easily separated.

Expression of oil

This is an extraction method mainly used for citrus oils. The oil is extracted by squeezing it out of sacs under the surface of the peel or skin of the fruit. At home the squeezing can be done by hand onto a clean sponge. Commercially oil is squeezed out of the peel by mechanical means, a process is called scarification.

Solvent method

The solvent method tends to be used to extract oil from the bark of trees, e.g., frankincense. Solvents such as alcohol or hydrocarbon are used to extract the essential oil, then the solvents are removed by distillation.

Enfleurage of oils

Petals or leaves are laid out on trays of wax or animal fat and crushed between wooden framed, glass trays. The plant matter is replaced regularly until the wax is saturated with essential oil. This method is used for the flower essences that are more delicate and difficult to obtain such as jasmine, neroli, and rose.

Using Essential Oils

The versatility of essential oils makes them one of nature's wonderful gifts. Essential oils contain the active ingredients of a plant in a highly concentrated and potent form. They need to be treated with care and should *never* be applied directly to the skin undiluted. However, there are a few exceptions to this rule, lavender being one of them such as for a skin burn. Essential oils are mixed with carrier oils, an aspect called blending that will be discussed later. There are many ways of utilising the fragrance and therapeutic properties of essential oils as follows:

Inhalation: Steam inhalation is an excellent method for treating respiratory problems (blocked sinus, colds, influenza etc.). Add 3 to 6 drops of an essential oil (tea tree or peppermint) to a bowl of steaming hot water. Place a towel over the head and breathe deeply. Keep adding more hot water as the water cools down.

Massage: Using the combined benefits of massage and essential oils is a wonderful way of triggering the body's natural healing ability. It will stimulate and cleanse the flow of blood and lymph fluid by entry through the skin. For every 10mls of carrier oil use a minimum of 3 drops and no more than a maximum of 10 drops of essential oil. Lavender, rosemary, and rose are all good therapeutic oils to use.

Diffusers: Fill the top of a china bowl diffuser with water and add a few drops of essential oil onto the surface. The candle in the pot underneath heats the water and slowly releases the natural fragrance into the air. Electric diffusers are available too which work at the flick of a switch.

Baths: Run your bath, then add the essential oil. Close the door of the bathroom so the aromatic vapour doesn't escape. Give the bath a good whisk with your hand before getting into it to ensure the oils are mixed with the water and not sitting in a little pool on top of the water. Soak for at least ten minutes, relaxing and breathing deeply. Use 5 to 10 drops of essential oil. For sensitive skin, it is best to dilute the oil in a base oil first.

Diffusers: Add 4 to 5 drops of essential oil to a large bowl or basin of hot water. To refresh tired feet, use peppermint, rosemary or thyme. To soothe aching feet try lavender oil.

Handbath: To soothe chapped or blistered skin, use 3 to 4 drops of essential oil of lavender in a bowl. Soak the blistered part in the bowl or bathe by applying the water to the affected area.

Shower: Wash as usual. Then add 1 or 2 drops of essential oil to your face cloth and rub it over yourself briskly as you continue to stand under the running water. Breathe in deeply as you do so. Eucalyptus, tea tree, lavender, and rose oil are all good oils to use in a shower. Spray full strength tea tree on the fungus of athletes foot. Avoid rubbing oil near your eyes and delicate tissues.

Sauna: In a sauna only use eucalyptus, tea tree, or pine essential oils. These oils enter the body with inhalation and exit through perspiration. They are excellent cleansers and de-toxifiers. Add 2 drops of essential oil to a cupful of water and splash it over the hot coals which will produce steam.

Jacuzzi or Spa: Add 10 to 15 drops essential oil to the jacuzzi or spa.

Room Sprays: To make a room spray blend 10 drops of essential oil to a cupful of water. An optional addition is to add a tablespoon of vodka or pure alcohol to preserve this mixture. Shake well. It can be sprayed in the air or on carpets, curtains etc. Be careful that the spray doesn't fall on wood because it could produce marks on wood. Eucalyptus, rosemary, and lavender are all good oils to use for room sprays.

Candles: 1 to 2 drops of essential oil for a candle. Light the candle and wait until the wax begins to melt, then add the oil to the melting wax. Be careful that it doesn't fall on the flame because essential oils are extremely flammable. Use a dropper to deliver the oil for safety.

Woodfires: Use one or two drops of essential oil on a log and leave for half an hour before lighting the fire. Once the fire gets going it will release your favourite aroma (these logs can be prepared ahead of time).

Hot Water Bowls: Put boiling water into a bowl and add 1 to 6 drops of essential oil. Close the doors and windows and allow 5 minutes for the aroma to penetrate the room.

Handkerchief: The ideal way to prevent winter chills and use for colds and influenza or even headaches. Place 3 or 4 drops onto a handkerchief and inhale. Eucalyptus, tea tree, and peppermint oils are popular and extremely useful during winter months as protection and treatment for coughs and colds.

Other ways

Above are only a few ways to use essential oils. You can add them to your shoe rack and in your shoes to deodorize shoes, also freshen up your wardrobe and clothes by adding a few drops to the bottom of your wardrobe.

For household cleaning, essential oils can be added to the water to effectively aid the cleaning process. For example, add lavender to your water and then wipe around the frames of your windows, this is a deterrent to the common housefly. Tea tree oil is an excellent antiseptic and a bactericidal as well as being anti-fungal and anti-viral, which makes it an excellent choice as part of your cleaning regime for the bathroom and toilet particularly if a member of the family is suffering from a gastric upset or infectious disease.

Base or Carrier oils

Base or carrier oils play an important role in diluting an essential oil because most pure essential oils are too highly concentrated to be used directly on the skin. The base oils will dilute the essential oil and allow the oil to spread evenly and easily over the skin. Also, a base oil will have its own therapeutic property and often encourages quick absorption of the essential oil. Always ask a person if they have any allergies to oils or fragrances. Also you would take care about which oils to use, i.e., if there is an allergy to peanuts, you would not use peanut oil.

Oils were mentioned in the section on massage, but we will explore them further here. Below is a list of some good base oils that are available to mix a blended oil. Table 3: Mixing Oils, provides a guideline for mixing base oils with essential oils.

Sweet Almond Oil, obtained from the almond kernel, is an excellent oil for many types of skin. It contains glycosides, minerals, vitamins and is very rich in protein. This oil is probably the best all-purpose carrier oil because it is both light and neutral. It is excellent for all skin types and helps relieve itching, soreness, dryness and inflammation of the skin. This oil can be used as a 100% base oil.

Apricot Oil obtained from apricot kernels contains minerals and vitamins and it is also good for all skin types, especially prematurely aged, sensitive, inflamed, and dry skins. It can be used as a 100% base oil.

Avocado Oil obtained from fruit is a thicker oil but very good for the skin too. It contains vitamins, protein, lecithin and fatty acids. It is especially good for dry, dehydrated skin and eczema. Use as a 10% dilution with 90% of another base oil.

Carrot Oil, an essential oil in its own right, is often used in base oils. It contains vitamins, minerals and beta-carotene. It is an oil that is beneficial for premature ageing, itchy, and dry, skin as well as for psoriasis and eczema. It aids in rejuvenation of the skin and reduces scarring. Use as a 10% dilution with 90% of another base oil.

Evening Primrose Oil contains gamma linoleic acid, vitamins and minerals. It can be used for pre-menstrual tension, multiple sclerosis, and menopausal problems as well as being an excellent oil for the treatment of psoriasis and eczema. Also, it helps to prevent premature ageing of the skin. Use as a 10% dilution with 90% of another base oil.

Olive Oil contains protein, minerals, and vitamins. It can be used in rheumatic conditions, hair care, and cosmetics and it is very soothing. Use as a 10% dilution with 90% of another base oil.

Peanut Oil contains protein, vitamins and minerals. It is suitable for all skin types and can be used as a 100% base oil. Useful for arthritic joints.

Safflower Oil contains protein, minerals and vitamins. It is suitable for all skin types and can be used as a 100% base oil.

Sesame Oil contains vitamins, minerals, proteins, lecithin and amino acids. It can be used for psoriasis, eczema, rheumatism, and arthritis. It is suitable for all skin types and is used as a 10% dilution with 90% of another base oil.

Soya bean oil contains vitamins and minerals. It is suitable for all skin types and can be used as a 100% base oil.

Sunflower oil contains vitamins and minerals. This is a light oil suitable for all skin types and can be used as a 100% base oil.

Wheat germ oil contains protein, minerals and vitamins. It can be used for eczema, psoriasis, and prematurely aged skin. It is suitable for all skin types. Use as a 10% dilution with 90% of another base oil.

Coconut oil is a nourishing skin oil but tends to solidify in the cold and become fluid in a warm environment.

If in any doubt about a person's sensitivity to an oil first test the oil on their forearm by placing a small patch and leaving it for 15 minutes. If there is a reaction, such as itchiness or redness wash off the oil with soap and water and don't use it.

Below is a chart showing guidelines for quantities to use when essential oils are mixed with base oils.

Table 3 Mixing Oils

Minimum essential oil	Maximum essential oil	Milliliters of base oil
0 drops	1 drop	1ml
2 drops	5 drops	5 mls
6 drops	15 drops	15 mls
8 drops	20 drops	20mls

*5mls equals 1 teaspoonful

Blending Oils

Because each essential oil has a particular fragrance and therapeutic property there is an art to blending essential oils with base (carrier) oils. Some oils mix well together others will overpower one another. For example, frankincense and ginger are both heavy smelling essences, which when combined together give an overpowering, unpleasant smell. Whereas lavender and rosemary will blend nicely together. In general, it is best to use a maximum of three oils in a blend. Each essential oil is described as either a top note, middle note, or base note. One of the traditional methods in aromatherapy is to create a blend using a synergy of a top, middle, or base note; this is the science and art of aromatherapy.

Top Note is usually the first scent you experience when smelling a blend.

Middle Note is the scent that last longer so this choice imparts the warmth and fullness of the blend.

Base Note is the heavy smelling scent which has a profound influence on the blend as a whole. Base notes tend to have a strong influence on the mental, emotional, and spiritual plane.

Examples of essential oil notes that blend well together are shown in Table 4.

Table 4: Blending Essential oil Notes

Top Note	Middle Note	Base Note
Basil	Chamomile	Clove
Eucalyptus	Geranium	Frankincense
Tea tree	Lavender	Sandalwood

Thyme	Peppermint	Cedar wood
Lemon	Rosemary	Ginger

There are no hard and fast rules in blending essential oils for home use, however, the suggestions in the table above will be useful. Until you have gained experience, do not blend more than three oils at a time. Start with one base oil plus one essential oil and you need not be concerned about whether the essential oil is top, middle, or base note. Oils used for massage therapy should be a pleasant-smelling blend and something that is therapeutic for the subject. Remember scent is a very personal experience and what might smell wonderful to you, may smell disgusting to someone else. When you create a blend, decide your purpose for creating it and ask your subject whether they like it or not. A blend for stress will be very different to a blend for an infection. The blend will always be mixed with a base carrier oil for use on the skin when doing massage.

Ensure that the subject does not have any allergies to either the base carrier oil or essential oil before using it on their skin. First ask, then if unsure rub a little of each of the oils you intend using on the subject's forearm as a test. If the oil patch becomes itchy or red, don't use it as they probably have some sensitivity or allergy to it. The most common allergy is to peanut oil. However, peanut oil, although a bit sticky is excellent to massage into arthritic joints.

The following essential oils are a good starting point if you are intending to use oils for healing. Ensure you do not keep essential oils near any homeopathic remedies because the subtle energy of homeopathic remedies will be affected by the overpowering vibrational energy of the essential oils. Keep essential oils in a separate wooden box or metal container in a cool place.

Lavender

Lavender is an all-time favorite – whether it is grown in the home garden and used as a tea, diffusion, or as an essential oil. No list of essential oils would be complete without including lavender. It is capable of so many important functions and is a delight to use. It is effective in the treatment of burns and scalds (pure essential oil), promotes healing, and prevents scarring. It also stimulates the immune system and contributes to the healing process by stimulating the cells of a wound to regenerate quickly. Lavender is also known to alleviate effects of shock. It can be used as a mood enhancer and anti-depressant. To most people it smells divine!

Lavender comes from the Roman word "lavare" which means to wash. In fact, this was one of the most favoured aromatics used by the Romans in their daily bathing rituals. Both the Greeks and Romans burned lavender twigs as a room purifier to ward off the plague, and lavender bags (small muslin bags filled with lavender flowers) have been placed in linen and clothes drawers for centuries to keep moths and insects away.

Ways to use Lavender

Sunburn – Mix 4 to 5 drops of Lavender oil with an aloe vera gel or with a cream and apply several times a day.

Burns – Small burns and scalds apply neat (undiluted), to the skin.

Bee & Wasp stings – Apply neat to the sting.

Physical and Nervous fatigue – Add to a bath, foot, or hand bath.

Insomnia – Apply one drop each side of the pillow. Use in a bath or footbath prior to retiring.

Headaches – Rub on temples and base of skull

Colds and Flu – Use as an inhalation

Summary of uses: Burns, inflammation, cuts, wounds, eczema, dermatitis, fainting, headaches, influenza, insomnia, hysteria, migraine, nausea, nervous tension, infections, bacterial conditions, sores, ulcers, acne, boils, asthma, rheumatism, arthritis.

Tea Tree

Tea Tree is anti-bacterial, anti-viral, and anti-fungal which makes it useful in a wide range of conditions.

Ways to use Tea Tree:

Acne – Use 1 to 2 drops in a face wash.

Nappy Rash –Add 1 drop to cream or ointment.

Chicken Pox Blisters

Add to the bath or mix the following together in a bottle:

- 7 drops of Tea Tree,

- 7 drops of Lavender,
- 50mls of Witch hazel,
- 50mls of Water.
- Use cotton wool swab or soft cotton ball and dab on the blisters.

Cold Sores (Herpes): Apply neat to the cold sores.

Ear Infections add together:

- 2 drops of Tea Tree oil
- 10 mls of Olive oil
- Soak a cotton wool plug or cotton swab in this mixture and insert gently into the ear.
- Alternatively, shake the bottle well (dropper bottle) and place a few drops directly into the ear then
- Plug the outer ear with a large soft cotton wool swab.

Athlete's Foot (Tinea) add together:

- 2 drops of Tea Tree
- 1 drop of Lavender
- Dip a cotton bud into the mixture and smear it between the toes and around the nails.

Vaginal Thrush (Candida): Add 2 drops to a cupful of warm water. Use as a douche, or soaked on a tampon. Four drops can be added to a bathtub.

Warts: Apply directly to warts using an earbud.

Brown age spots on hands: 1 drop tea tree to 20 mls glycerine.

Summary of Uses – Fungal infections, thrush, nappy rash, viral and bacterial infections, colds, influenza, ear infections, cold sores, warts, acne, age spots.

Peppermint

Peppermint is an excellent oil for most body systems – it aids digestion, helps alleviate respiratory problems, and improves the circulation. It is anti-inflammatory and antiseptic. Within its range of uses peppermint is an excellent repellent for mice, fleas, and ants.

Ways to use Peppermint:

Travel Sickness - Add 1 to 2 drops of essential oil of peppermint to a tissue or handkerchief and sniff. You can add 1 to 2 drops to a cotton wool ball and place in the ear.

Stomach pain and colic - Make a compress with 1 or 2 drops of peppermint oil and place over the stomach or make a massage oil and apply to the stomach area in an anti-clockwise direction.

Tired feet - Add some peppermint oil to a footbath, wonderful for tired, smelly, feet.

Hot flushes - Make a cold water compress with two drops of peppermint oil to relieve hot flushes.

Sinusitis: Make an inhalation with 3 drops of peppermint and 3 drops of lavender, and then inhale.

Mental fatigue, headaches, and migraine: 2 to 3 drops as an inhalation or use an oil diffuser in the room.

Arthritis: Add 10 drops of essential oil to 10mls base oil (peanut is excellent) and massage into joints.

Summary of uses: Inflammation, nausea, indigestion, fevers, flatulence, headaches, migraines, and arthritis.

Eucalyptus

Eucalyptus is most commonly known for its therapeutic properties relating to chest problems and cold symptoms. It is a wonderfully versatile oil because it is anti-inflammatory, antiseptic, antibiotic, diuretic and deodorising.

Ways to use Eucalyptus:

Colds and Sinus – One of the best ways to use eucalyptus oil is through an inhalation by adding 6 drops of eucalyptus to a bowl of boiling water. Place a towel over the head and breathe in the steam.

Chest Rub - To make a chest rub add 5 drops of eucalyptus and a dessert spoon of base oil. Other oils that can be safely added to this mixture are 2 drops each of tea tree, rosemary, and thyme.

Fever – To reduce fever add 8 drops to the bathtub.

Baths – By adding eucalyptus to your bathtub, it can help relieve many ailments. Helps with muscular/ rheumatic aches and pains, relieves cystitis, any infection, reduces fever, and will also clear the head.

Summary of uses: Sore throats, coughs, bronchitis, sinusitis, skin infections, ulcers, sores, rheumatism, aches and pains, as an antiseptic and anti-inflammatory.

Geranium

The essential oil of geranium is extracted from a species of geranium called Pelargonium. It is an oil that works profoundly on the emotions as well as being useful during influenza epidemics.

Ways to use Geranium:

Infections of the throat and mouth – 1 drop of Geranium and 1 drop of Tea Tree oil, add to half a glass of warm water. Gargle, but be careful not to swallow.

Influenza – add 6 drops geranium to a bath or use 3 drops in a room diffuser.

Improvement of circulation to the legs – Add 3 drops of geranium and 2 drops of rosemary to 10mls of carrier oil. Massage into the legs.

Insect Repellent – Add to a carrier oil of your choice and rub on to the skin.

Jetlag – Have a bath with 3 drops of geranium and 2 drops of rosemary, to feel wide awake.

Chilblains – Add 3 drops to a footbath.

Nervous tension and depression – Use any of the above.

Summary of uses: Geranium is unusual in that it is both a sedative as well as a mood enhancer and this makes it an invaluable remedy when treating nervous tension and depression as well as emotional problems associated with menstrual and menopausal problems. Also useful for diarrhoea, diabetes, influenza, circulation, skin problems, frostbite, and jet lag. Its antiseptic and astringent properties contribute to its general usefulness.

Rosemary

Rosemary is steeped in history, folklore and tradition. Long ago, Greeks and Romans twined rosemary in their hair in the belief that it would quicken their mind and improve their memory. Rosemary was considered the herb of fidelity and was often an ingredient in the cup passed at weddings. Rosemary was scattered on the floor of homes so that its fragrance would cover up foul smells. It was also thought to have disinfectant properties.

Some ways to use Rosemary:

Hair and Scalp - Add 2 drops of rosemary into water for the final hair rinse as a conditioner.

Mixture for head lice:

- 25 grams of beeswax
- 50mls of castor oil.
- Two drops of each rosemary, geranium, and lavender.
- Melt the beeswax over a pot of boiling water.
- Add the castor oil until a creamy consistency is achieved.
- Cool.
- Add the essential oils while stirring.
- Rub well into the scalp and leave overnight.

Sports massage/aching muscle blend:

- Add 3 drops of rosemary, 1 drop of eucalyptus, 1 drop of lavender,
- Add 10mls of carrier oil,
- Blend well.

Headaches and Fatigue - add 2 drops of rosemary to a handkerchief and inhale.

Circulation and memory - Add 3 drops to an air diffuser. Apply to skin as a perfume.

Summary of uses: Stimulates circulation and memory. Useful for gout, headaches, fatigue, rheumatism, skin infections, muscular aches and pains, sprains, and as an analgesic.

Thyme

Thyme has wonderful anti-viral, antibiotic, antiseptic, and diuretic properties. Essential oil of Thyme should be used with great care and must be used in moderation. It should never be applied to the skin undiluted and *do not use it with small children*. The ancient Egyptians incorporated thyme in their embalming fluids and Greeks drank an herbal infusion of the leaves after a meal to aid digestion. The English have always used thyme for flavouring and aiding digestion of food.

Summary of uses: Helps fatigue and anxiety, but it is best known as a natural antiseptic for treating coughs and infections of the respiratory tract. Use in a diffuser or bathtub and it will assist in the elimination of toxic wastes from the body. Other conditions include whooping cough, warts, rheumatism, neuralgia, fatigue and acne. Just to make it a perfect all-rounder, thyme will discourage all manner of parasites and insects from invading your home. Wipe around window sills with thyme oil wherever you observe them entering into the house.

Lemon

Early seafarers stocked up with fresh lemons before a long sea voyage to help prevent scurvy and to purify the ships drinking water. It has astringent and antiseptic properties and is useful in the first aid kit to treat cuts, bruises, and insect's bites. Lemon has a wide range of uses and an essential oil of lemon can be used in many ways.

Some ways to use Lemon:

Nose Bleed: Lie on your back, pinch the tip of nostrils and inhale from a tissue infused with 3 drops of lemon oil.

Constipation: To a glass of water add 3 drops of lemon oil and drink. Also, into carrier oil add 10 drops of lemon oil and massage small circles in a clockwise direction over the lower stomach area, up to three times a day.

Hay Fever: Place 1 drop of lemon oil onto a tissue and inhale throughout the day.

Liver and Gall Bladder: Add 1 drop essential oil of lemon to a glass of water and make this your first drink in the morning. Add one drop of lemon oil to one tablespoonful of olive oil. Take three times a day for three days each month for 3 months as a liver and gall bladder cleanser.

Summary of uses:

Lowers blood pressure, for colds, digestive problems, fever, gallstones, and nervous conditions, as a liver tonic, astringent, and antiseptic. Use in skin care preparations for oily skin. Also useful as a water purifier and insect repellent.

If you find you have an affinity for essential oils, there is so much more to study in this field. This chapter is only a small sample to encourage you to begin experimenting and discovering the amazing world of aromatherapy.

CHAPTER ELEVEN

Massage

Hands are for Healing

Most people enjoy and benefit from massage. Our hands provide a means of healing when used with a loving intent. Massage is an excellent home-help treatment to share with a partner, friends, or family member. This chapter will teach you some basic knowledge about massage but is not intended to provide enough knowledge for you to become a qualified massage practitioner.

Massage has been practiced by human beings throughout the world for thousands of years. Ancient records and writings reveal that massage was used before either medicine or allied sciences, as we know them today, were even understood. Early references to massage came from Kong Fu, and Chinese books of uncertain date but thought to have been written about 3000 B.C. There are references to massage in sacred books of the Hindu religion, and also in very early historical writings from Egypt, Persia, the Roman Empire, and Ancient Greece. Many cultures and traditions show well-developed systems of hands on healing.

Homer referred to the benefits of the art in his epic poem the *Odyssey*. (believed to be composed about the 8th century BC)[54]. He records that beautiful women rubbed their heroes with oils and thus were able to ease the fatigue of exhausted warriors. Herodicus, a famous Greek physician (5th century BC), insisted that all his patients were to benefit from a good diet and massage using beneficial herbs and oils. About that time the

Gymnasia became established throughout Greek provinces and massage became associated with health and sports. He specified that massage should begin with slow and gentle rubbing working into a faster and deeper technique followed by gentle friction. He was believed to be one of Hippocrates tutors.[55]

Hippocrates (born around 460 BC) believed in the healing power of nature and the fact that the body if given the opportunity could heal itself. He was one of the first to make scientific studies about massage.[56] Hippocrates recommended friction for sprains and abdominal massage for constipation – also he valued massage work in acute illness and many forms of paralysis, rheumatism, and obesity. He was observant enough to note the direction that massage should take for best effects in the respective ailments. This was particularly clever because it was about 1800 to 2000 years later that any real knowledge of the circulatory system was understood.

Like several other arts, massage had its golden eras, and at other times, its reputation sank, this appeared to happen in the Middle Ages. In the 18th century, massage started to regain its degree of power and application, especially in Europe by medical men. Professor Henry Ling (1776 - 1839), a Swede, was a brilliant man who developed another branch of massage. He taught fencing and gymnastics and by studying the work of previous gymnasts, he made a scientific ruling, or classification, of all movements of the body, as passive, active or resisted movements. Today we have *Swedish Massage* named after his work.

Massage is a method of supporting the flow of fluid through the body. The action of massage techniques can stimulate blood and lymph flow and assist in the excretion of waste products. Massage will release tension in tissues, particularly muscles and nerves, and generate relaxation and relief from stress and anxiety. Massage can compensate, in part, for lack of exercise and disuse of muscles in persons who, because of injury, illness, or age, are forced to remain inactive.

Massage is given in many ways for widely different purposes. Relaxation massage is generally administered through the practitioner's hands. Mechanical massage instruments are available and useful, but when human hands come into contact with a subject something very different happens to the recipient. The person giving a massage, through their caring attitude, can enhance feelings of wellbeing in the recipient and often in return will feel uplifted as well.

Skillful working massage hands depend upon the dedication of the practitioner and development of hand sensitivity that can probe and discover tension in muscles and discern the source of pain. Those hands can become both relaxing and soothing instruments to soothe pain and release tension from the body of the recipient and enable healing to occur. When a practitioner is working with their hands, they are working as a 'living instrument' – just like 'living water' there is a difference. The human body is 70% water, and works as an electrical conductor, therefore the positive thoughts and intent of the person giving a massage will have a healing effect on the recipient.

It is not possible in this book to provide a full instructional course about massage, but the basic massage movements will be described so you can practice them on yourself, a partner, or family members at home. Always ask your subject for feedback when you perform the strokes. Ask if your hand techniques are too soft, too hard, too fast, too slow, or just right for them.

You can perform self-massage on your own hands, arms, feet, legs, face, chest and abdomen quite easily and you may even reach your shoulders comfortably. If you find another person interested in massage, then practice on each other and give reciprocal massages. Children love massage (if they are not too ticklish) and are often keen to learn too.

There are five fundamental movements in Swedish massage. These techniques can be adapted for use on various parts of the body:

1. Effleurage (stroking);
2. Friction (deep, fast rubbing);
3. Petrissage (kneading, compression)
4. Tapotement (percussion);
5. Vibrations (shaking & trembling).

The above are common terms used for massage movements with a brief self-explanatory definition. The first three strokes, i.e. effleurage, friction, and petrissage can be practiced on yourself in the shower. Lather your hands well with soap and start with your arms and legs. The usual order of massage movements is to begin with effleurage, next friction, then either superficial or deeper kneading, followed by tapotement and vibration. Effleurage and petrissage are the two most popular strokes and you may decide to focus only on these movements. It is good to start and finish a massage with effleurage. Heavier strokes are always towards the heart.

For a massage of the head, neck, shoulders, arms, feet or legs, the person to be massaged (recipient) may sit on a chair or stool. When massaging the arm, it should rest upon a table or support. In massaging the leg and foot, the recipient sits opposite the operator. When the abdomen, chest, back, or thighs, are to be massaged the recipient should lie on a bed, a suitable massage table, or a mat on the floor. A massage can take from 10 minutes to an hour or more depending upon how much of the body is to be massaged.

Always ensure the recipient is warm and comfortable before starting the massage and kept warm during the massage. Keep the parts of the body that are not being massaged covered with towels or a blanket for warmth and modesty. Provide enough pillows for comfort too.

Contraindications to massage

- The abdomen should not be massaged immediately after a meal.
- Where there is inflammation or pain, these places should be massaged very lightly or not massaged at all.
- *Never massage anyone with blood clots in their leg* or where a clot is likely to move into the blood stream.
- Older people have delicate skin so be very careful when giving massage to the elderly, some elderly people bruise easily.
- In chronic disease, such as diabetes and neurological problems, tissues may be damaged using strong massage techniques.
- Anyone with lack of feeling in their toes and feet, require extremely gentle treatment.
- Massaging a person with cancer is controversial; I believe the healing touch of a caring person may be what the individual needs when stressed and struggling with this illness.
- Limiting a massaging to the hands and feet can still be therapeutic for some of the above conditions.

Always use common sense - *if in doubt leave it out and don't do it!*

People have their own pain tolerance level. Some people like or require a firmer massage, while others need or want a much lighter touch. Gaining feedback from the recipient is important. Always ask the subject if your pressure is all right. "How is my pressure? Would you like me to go lighter/deeper? Are you comfortable?" It requires repeated practice to judge the correct amount of pressure for each person when doing a massage. It is better to err on the side of caution and cause no harm. Observe and listen to the subject in order to adjust the massage to suit the individual.

The strength of the various hand techniques is one of the principal points in applying massage treatment well. The hand must be gentle yet sufficiently firm in order to accomplish the desired results. As a rule, begin with gentle to moderate pressure, ascertain tolerance level and flow through into their comfort zone.

Contrary to popular belief deep massage is *not good* for athletes, after vigorous exercise, or after playing a game. Slow gentle movements are best using an appropriate cream or oil.

How to apply Effleurage/Stroking

Effleurage movements may be done with the lightest touch using tips of the fingers, or with the whole surface of the hand held in different ways. This is a soothing, relaxing movement. Various degrees of pressure can be used. They are generally long, flowing strokes that always begin the work in a particular body region. The easiest places to begin practice with these strokes are on the back, the legs, and arms.

Firmer pressure should be in the direction of the venous blood and lymph flow therefore, limbs are massaged more firmly in an upwards direction towards the center of the body. This is a general guide only and there are exceptions to the rule such as strokes on the head, face, feet, and hands. Do what you intuitively feel is right.

Hands are not lifted at the end of an effleurage stroke, but glide back to where they started, without pressure and without losing contact with the recipient. The following are several ways to do this movement:

❖ The fingers are held straight and close together, but not stiffly. The tips, or cushions, of the finger pads are placed on the part to be worked, e.g. the wrist - a straight upward stroke is made with little pressure, the fingers glide back with no pressure, do this about twenty times. This form of effleurage is useful at the beginning of a massage session.

❖ The cushions of the fingers are placed in the same way as the previous movement and then moved in overlapping circles, lightly and slowly moving on gradually without pressure. This is useful in insomnia (inability to sleep) performed along the spine, on the forehead, and over the head area.

❖ A straight stroke with the whole surface of the hand held flat, gliding back with the return stroke as before. This stroke is useful for larger body parts.

❖ The thumb is separated from the fingers and placed across the top of a limb, fingers are underneath, the limb held in the hand and strokes performed as before. This is a good way to effleurage the limbs of a child. With a child, one hand holds the small limb, and every aspect of it is done at the same time. This technique is also used on the inner and outer parts of large limbs.

❖ The hands are placed one on each side of a limb, fairly firm pressure is made upwards, both hands acting at the same time. This is similar to petrissage (kneading) and is useful in cases of obesity.

❖ The thumbs are placed parallel on top of a limb, the fingers underneath. A sweeping upward movement is made with each hand alternately, gliding back almost to the starting point, again sweeping upwards and back until the body part is covered.

❖ The knuckles of hands are used in the same manner to stroke large areas such as thighs.

How to apply Petrissage/Kneading or Compression

Petrissage is a much deeper movement than effleurage and performed mainly on muscles. Muscles are grasped between the thumbs and fingers or in the palms of the hands and kneaded, rolled, pressed, and squeezed by one or more of the following methods to stimulate circulation and lymph flow:

❖ Using the thumb and index finger, any single muscle or group of small muscles such as the cheek or the palm of the hand are grasped. The finger is kept steady and the muscle is rolled back onto it with the thumb, or the thumb is kept steady and the muscle is rolled back with the finger. Repeat several times - say five - then make a very slight onward movement. Repeat the kneading movement in the next area while maintaining contact.

❖ A group of muscles is grasped between the fingers and thumbs of both hands, the fingers being on one side and the thumbs on the other side; the thumbs are kept steady, and the muscle is worked back against them with the fingers or vice versa. Repeat on the same spot five times, move slightly onward and repeat.

❖ Grasp the muscles in the hand between the fingers and the heel of the hand or the ball of the thumb. Knead by using the heel of the hand against the fingers.

❖ Where there are masses of muscles such as in the arm or leg, grasp the muscles between the hands, one on each side, the fingers are kept steady, while the thumbs and palms work against them with an upward, outward, and spiral movement, in this way the tissues are rolled, squeezed, and kneaded. Every part of the operators hand must be kept in close contact with the muscles, then progress gradually upward. This is the deepest movement.

❖ A 'wringing' movement which is particularly effective on children whereby a limb is grasped in both hands, one in front of the other, very much as a wet cloth is held when being wrung out: the hands are twisted round the limb, backwards and forwards, carrying the muscles with them. The muscle is actually turned on the bone - both hands move in the same direction, which is then reversed. Care should be taken not to use too much pressure and 'jerking' movements must be avoided.

❖ Pincement is the name used to describe a petrissage movement where the muscles are not actually worked on as above, only the skin and the immediate underlying tissue is worked. The tissues are taken up between the fingers and thumbs, the fingers on one side, the thumbs on the other, held end to end. The thumbs work alternatively in rotatory manner and press and squeeze the tissues against the fingers. It is a useful movement to use for obese and oedematous (fluid filled) tissues, or conversely, with an extremely thin person, where muscles are wasted.

How to apply Friction

This movement may be performed with the thumbs, tips of the fingers, or palms of the hand. It consists of deep circular movements toward the center of a joint or around joints. It is often used over one group of muscles at a time. The tips of the fingers are generally used around the joints: and in the case of the knee joint, the ball of the thumb may be used. Apply five to ten circles on a spot, and then move on. Friction using the whole hand is effective on larger surfaces of the body. The purpose of friction is to limber up joints, tendons and muscles, to heat up tissues and to break up deposits in the tissues to facilitate their removal and reduce scar tissue.

Friction is always followed by effleurage. When working on an area, apply five to ten circular movements followed immediately by effleurage, then friction again, then effleurage, and so on.

How to apply Tapotement/Percussion

Tapotement is carried out by rapidly and rhythmically striking the body with the hands or the fingers in various positions. These percussion movements are from the wrist and are short and quick. The hands are raised not too far from the recipient's body. It is a light, sharp, rapid, springy movement, with the hands swinging from the wrists to stimulate tissues and is carried out in different ways, as follows:

- ❖ Slapping – this movement is carried out with the palm surface of the fingers which are held straight and close together. Make strike movements across the muscles, evenly and rhythmically, moving backward and forward, and in every direction, leaving no part untouched. This is a stimulating movement and does not need a lot of pressure behind it. Though slapping sounds harsh adjust your technique to make it acceptable to the recipient.
- ❖ Flail – this movement is carried out with the back of the semi-flexed fingers. Hold fingers loose and open and strike the body as

in the previous movement. These two movements are useful on the forearm, legs and back.

❖ Tapping – this movement is carried out with the tips of the open fingers, and all of the fingertips are used. It is suitable for the head and chest. Another application is with the tips brought together forming a cone. The cone is used on the thighs, over masses of muscles, or over fatty tissue.

❖ Beating – this movement is carried out with the outside border of the hand closed into a fist. Either using one hand or, applying both hands (alternately), strike the body applying the little finger side of the fist. It is used on the thighs and buttocks.

❖ Chopping or Hacking - this movement is carried out using the outside borders of the fingers which are separated and held loosely. Let the fingers fall together onto the body and allow the hands to strike the body alternately. As the strike occurs the little and third fingers come down together. It is generally used on the back muscles.

❖ Cupping – this movement is performed with the whole palmar surface of the hands. The palms are contracted so as to form a hollow or cup. The cupped hands strike the body alternately and is generally performed on the thighs and back.

Tapotement stimulates capillary and lymph circulation and nerves. Tapotement is excellent to use in atrophied (wasted) conditions of muscles because it increases contraction of muscle fibers and stimulates muscle contraction.

How to apply Vibration

Firmly place and fix the hand or fingers upon the recipient's body then produce a rapid shaking, trembling, vibrating movement. Vibrations come through the whole arm and foreman of the practitioner which is held straight. The hand does not do the work as it is held firmly in place on the skin of the recipient's body. The vibrating hand should occasionally be moved from place to place so that this shaking trembling sensation is conveyed to other parts of the recipient's body. The movements are even, elastic, and very rapid; the amount of pressure varies, but the hand is firmly held on the recipient's skin and does not slip or move across the skin at all. This is a difficult technique to master and there are variations as follows:.

❖ The fingers, drawn together at the tips, are placed on a particular spot; the arm and hand of the operator is made to tremble, and thus convey vibrations to the recipient. The fingers remain stationary.

❖ The fingers, separated from each other, are made to surround a joint and vibration conveyed to the joint in the same manner as above.

❖ The palm of one hand (or both hands) is placed on the abdomen (liver, stomach or intestines) or lung area. Vibration is applied. This is an excellent technique to loosen phlegm in the chest and to help the recipient cough it up.

❖ Knuckles or thumbs placed on each side of the spinal column. Slowly move up the spine area.

❖ Vibration is of value in stimulating the circulation, the glandular system, the nervous system, lungs, liver, and the movement of the bowels.

Whereabouts on the body do I start the massage?

If you are doing self-massage your hands and arms are the best place to start in order to try out the different massage techniques. Next try your feet and legs and then chest and abdomen. Begin practicing the first three strokes in the shower. Lather your hands well with soap or shower gel (called the medium) so they get slippery and start – use more medium and water as required.

After you have tried the techniques on yourself find a willing subject and practice the techniques on their back, legs and arms - then it's up to you to pace yourself and enjoy the experience. Start small then extend yourself as you become more at ease with the techniques and working without allowing your hands to get tired.

If you cannot find a subject, practice your techniques on a pillow or a large teddy bear until you find a willing subject.

Oils for Massage

There are several different kinds of products available to apply while doing massage these will help hands and fingers to slide over the recipient's skin. It is not absolutely necessary to use oils for massage – water is probably the most readily available and cheapest source of medium to use and you will be surprised how effective it is to use. Whether you use water, wax, cream, lotion, powder, or oil is up to you to decide what suits you and your recipient best.

One of the most economic massage oils is to use a light cooking oil such as sunflower oil and add a few drops of an essential oil such as oil of lavender (very relaxing) or rosemary (for muscles). Also, if you grow lavender or rosemary you could make your own lavender oil (or any other flower or herb oil). Of course, there are always more expensive and exotic massage oils, waxes, and creams that can be purchased if desired.

To Make a Massage oil at home (This is not an essential oil)

- Fill a jar with lavender flowers, leaves, and stalks.
- Cover lavender in the jar with sunflower oil or any other light oil.
- Leave in the sun, or a warm place, for two weeks.
- Strain and drain off the oil.
- Now use it for massage.

Exercises for the hands

When you first begin to perform massage techniques your hands and fingers may feel awkward and stiff. Therefore, it is a good idea to exercise your hands and fingers every day. Use every method possible to strengthen your fingers as you go about your daily tasks. Finger exercises will benefit your hands and strengthen them, so they won't be tired when doing massage. Flexible and fit fingers will be more relaxed and able to apply correct movements for whatever time is needed to complete a massage. If your hands are getting tired while applying massage techniques then slow down your pace, vary your techniques, and perform some effleurage movements between techniques which will relax and rest your hands.

Suggestions to strengthen your fingers and hands:

- Play a musical instrument to keep fingers flexible, e.g. piano, guitar, or ukulele.

- Take a heavy stick whirl it in alternate directions rapidly with a partly bent elbow.
- Place both hands on a table, palms downwards, allow your body weight to be taken up by the wrist, and then raise individually each finger slowly and as high as possible - one at a time - then slowly lower each finger with pressure. If this exercise is done correctly it is rather difficult, but it is extremely effective in strengthening the fingers.
- Spread the fingers as wide as possible, then slowly, firmly and with power of strength, open them further and stretch as far as possible. Close and repeat. The slower and stronger this exercise is done the better.
- Make bread, by kneading the dough with your hands, or work your hands making children's play dough.
- Massage your own hands during the day.

Always ensure when doing massage that your body is positioned comfortably. Stand or sit in the most comfortable position so that you do nor injure yourself.

Massage at Home

The above lessons are intended for persons using massage at home to sustain wellness; it in no way means that you are a now a professional massage practitioner. Professional massage practitioners require more training, they are required to abide by a Code of Ethics, and have rules about how to maintain a clinical practice. Although when working with massage at home you are not bound by any rules you need to always ensure the comfort of your subject, keep parts of their body warm that you are not working on by using towels, drapes, or blankets and respect modesty.

Now that you have the basic techniques it's up to you to practice and apply them effectively and safely. Everyone develops their own style and manner of procedure for doing massage and there will be variations between people because we are all individuals. The information provided here is a starting point for those seeking knowledge about the wonderful hands on therapy called massage. Children love to be massaged and can easily be taught these techniques too.

Always use common sense and *if in doubt then don't do it until you have a professional opinion as to whether massage would be helpful or not.*

Now that you have the basic techniques to perform massage movements develop your own style and enjoy the journey!

Hands were designed for helping and a caring touch is therapeutic

CHAPTER TWELVE

Foot Therapy

*Feet are the foundation for the body. Fix the foundation and
you regenerate the body, enliven the soul, and step forward
into a new day, renewed, vibrant, and energised.*

Foot Therapy in the Home

Feet are an incredible part of the human body. In this chapter various ways
to work on feet in order to improve health and sustain wellness will be
described. The feet are an accessible part of the body and applying a few
techniques to the feet is an excellent non-threatening way to give hands
on treatment to children, family, and friends. In fact, at home the giver
and receiver can both participate at the same time. Methods discussed are
firstly, Zone Therapy, which was a term used before foot therapy developed
into the profession of Reflexology. Secondly, another useful technique as
it relates to foot therapy is the Metamorphic Technique.

Reflexology

Reflexology grew out of zone therapy and is a whole range of treatments
working on either the feet, hands, ears, or any part of the body within a
specific zone. Here, we describe some basic techniques that can be used
on the feet at home yet in no way intends to train you in the profession
of reflexology. Introducing you to foot techniques will enable you to help

yourself, your family, and friends to be healthy and well. Our focus will be to recognize zones on the feet that will effectively treat other parts of the body.

Reflexology has grown in popularity and is now integrated into the practice of many nurses, physiotherapists, naturopaths, and massage therapists around the world as an adjunct to their conventional and complementary treatments. Reflexology is a profession of its own nowadays, and students are trained to a very high standard before graduating and going into clinical practice.[57]

Zone Therapy

Zone Therapy applies what is known as the stimulus/reflex principle to health and healing through foot reflexes. It has been suggested that reflex responses enable the secretion of endorphins and other natural chemicals within the body that encourage tissues to relax and heal. Zone Therapy on the feet appears to activate a 'gate control mechanism' that reduces the perception of pain. There is also evidence that zone therapy on the feet leads to healing throughout the body. In this manner, the whole body is treated – the function of the body improves, energy increases, and wellness results.

Zone Therapy on the feet improves circulation and elimination throughout the body. Through stimulation of foot reflexes, nutrients and oxygen are delivered to the area being treated through the blood supply, and waste material flows back into the general circulation for excretion through the kidneys and other excretory organs. Major plexuses for the lymph system are also located in the feet and zone therapy techniques stimulate lymphatic movement as well.

The idea of stimulating reflexes of the feet to heal and sustain health is not foreign to many cultures. Knowledge about zones and reflexes within the body can be found in writings and inscriptions from ancient Chinese, Egyptian, English and European cultures. Ancient people knew the value of walking bare footed over rocky ground and twigs in the forests to stimulate reflexes in the feet that benefited the whole body. A western medical doctor, Dr. William Fitzgerald, is acknowledged as the founder of Zone Therapy and he was responsible for bringing his findings to the attention of his colleagues.

A graduate of the University of Vermont Dr. Fitzgerald first worked at Boston City Hospital, then went on to become a member of staff at the Central London Nose and Throat Hospital. Upon his return to the USA and while the chief surgeon in the Nose and Throat department of St Francis Hospital, Hartford, he demonstrated the value of 'Zone Therapy' to his medical colleagues which he believed was an excellent form of treatment. His colleagues were not particularly interested in this new method of Zone Therapy, so Dr. Fitzgerald focused upon educating the public in self-help methods. He frequently encouraged his patients to clutch wooden or metal combs firmly in their hands several times a day. This had an energizing effect on their whole body as it worked on their reflexes. He observed that sick people improved from an array of different illnesses and this work was the starting point for documenting reflexology. *Zone Therapy*[58] was the first Western book to describe the application of pressure on one part of the body in order to relieve symptoms in another part of the body. Fitzgerald provided a model for zone therapy showing that the body is divided into ten equal zones – each zone linked to corresponding body parts and organs of the body. He demonstrated that working within a zone on one part of the body had a beneficial effect on another part of the body in the same zone.

Zones of the Body

The following diagram (Fig. 3) illustrates the ten zones of the body reflected in the feet.

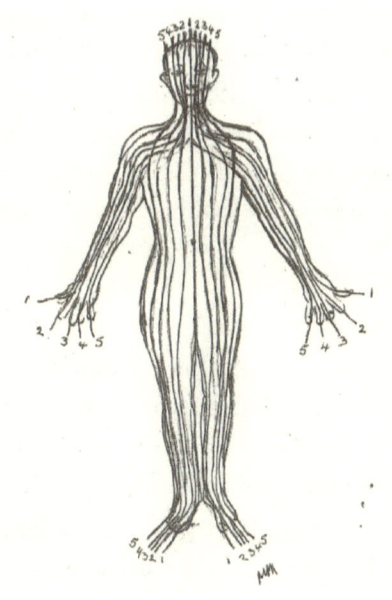

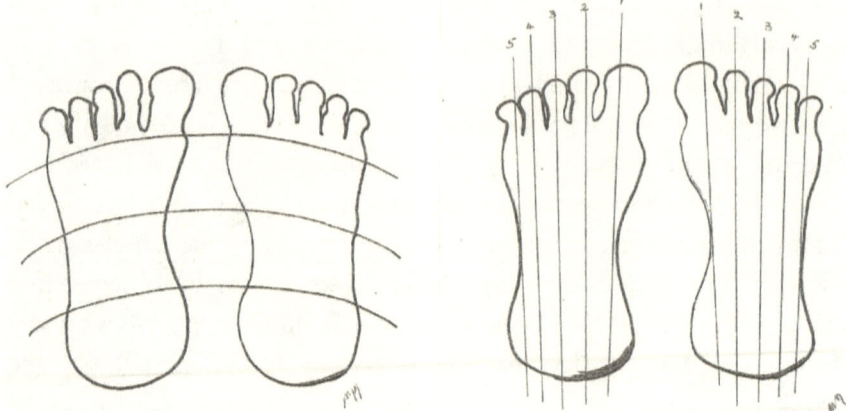

Figure 3: The Ten Zones of the Body Reflected in the Feet

In the USA during the 1930's, Eunice Ingham came across Fitzgerald's methods while working as a therapist for Dr. Joseph Riley. She began to use these zone therapy techniques (which did not require medical training) on the hands and feet - particularly on the feet. She discovered that discomfort in the soles of the feet varied according to the individual and their state of health. Eunice Ingham began calling her version of zone therapy 'Reflexology' and promoted it as a 'science and art'. Eunice Ingham taught many natural therapists and others her reflexology techniques. Ingham based her work on Fitzgerald's methods, then experimented with her own techniques and after carrying out further research published her books, *Stories the Feet Can Tell* (1932), along with its sequel, *Stories the Feet Have Told.* [59] These books have been read and used widely by natural health practitioners and the general public and have no doubt been the inspiration for others to teach, research, practice and write further about reflexology.

Zone Therapy and Reflexology Charts
Today there are a number of different zone therapy and reflexology charts that show relationships from areas on the feet to body parts and organs. The simplistic diagrams (Figure 3) provide an idea about how to visualize body parts located from reflexes on the feet. First visualize the body divided into five longitudinal parts on each foot going from the foot up to the head. Between each vertical line are located parts of the

148

body that can be treated in a reflex manner from the feet. Next visualize three transverse lines going across each foot. Above the first line are zones related to the head and neck areas of the body. Above the second line are zones related to organs of the chest area. Above the third line are zones for the abdominal organs mainly related to digestion. Below the third line are organs and tissues related to the lower part of the body. Between each vertical line are located parts of the body between the lines.

Zone therapy is an excellent method to facilitate natural changes and healing within the body as you allow the body to heal itself. This therapy will assist the body to self-heal and sustain wellness.

Contraindications for zone therapy

Extreme care is required when treating the feet of a diabetic, or anyone who has neurological problems with loss of feeling or loss of sensation in their feet. Also, although no harm can be done, corns and bunions can be painful and may need to be avoided. Always use common sense and if feet are off limits then you can always do zone therapy on hands or any other part of the body in the related zone. For example, if a knee joint is painful you could work on an elbow.

Techniques for foot therapy

Whole hands, pads of fingers, thumbs, and the knuckle of a bent finger, are all choices to use when applying techniques to a foot. These techniques can be used as a self-help treatment or to help another. Ensure you have short fingernails before starting.

Sweeping technique

Apply sweeping movements over the whole foot with one or both hands. This is a good technique to start and finish a session. This movement is likened to the effleurage or stroking movement of massage.

Circular technique

Apply pads of the fingers and thumbs to create a gentle to firm circular motion. Work on the same spot then move along, overlapping each section so that the whole area is covered. Use this technique on the bottom, sides, and top of each foot.

Caterpillar walk (crawl)

- Apply finger or thumb and start by positioning the finger at a 45- degree angle to the foot.
- Roll the hand forward so the finger comes to a right angle with the foot.
- The finger stays in the same place, but the rolling movement creates more pressure on the point.
- Crawl like a caterpillar along the foot with the finger by moving slightly forward with the finger then slightly backwards with the hand.
- Roll the hand forward again, as before, until the finger comes to a right angle once again.
- Repeat with pressure, come back, and then move onward again.
- This technique is best used on the bottom of the foot, working from heel to toe, up the longitudinal zones of the foot.
- Next work on the transverse sections across the foot (thumb is usually easier to apply across the foot) until the whole foot has been covered.

Rock and roll

- Bend first finger of the working hand and tuck the first part of it into the thumb.
- Using the flat part of the bent finger, between first and second knuckle, and rock and roll along the bottom of the foot.
- As you roll onto the second knuckle a little extra pressure can be used to effectively add pressure to the knuckle point so that it can go deep into an area of the foot if necessary.
- Be systematic and sensitive to the needs of the recipient as you cover the whole foot.

Use of Water, Powder, Oils and Creams

To facilitate a smooth treatment, you may choose to use water, powder, oil, cream – or nothing at all except bare hands. Water or powder are both very slippery yet are sometimes convenient when that's all there is available. Oils and creams are less slippery, are nice to work with, and help hands move smoothly as well as being good for any dry skin of the subject, and hands of the practitioner.

Applying the Foot Therapy technique

- Start with a comfortable position for both you and the subject.
- Soak the feet for five minutes or wash them in a basin of warm water.
- Dry the feet.
- Cover the right foot up with a small towel and start working on the other foot.
- Take the left foot into both hands and hold in a caring manner for a moment then make a sweeping movement along the whole foot.
- Repeat the sweeping movement a few times. This gentle caring start to the session helps the subject relax and suggests the start of something enjoyable.
- Begin your session with circular movements and caterpillar technique using fingers and/or thumbs and work up through each zone from the base of the foot to the top of the toes.
- Repeat 3 times.
- During this time note where sore points are and whether you feel any 'gritty' deposits beneath the surface. These are the areas you will come back to and work on further with the rock and roll technique.
- When you begin to work with reflexes don't do it for too long, particularly if areas are very sore and sensitive to touch.
- Ten minutes for each foot is a good starting time.
- Any tenderness in the foot will disappear as body function improves and pressure on any tender spot will become much more pleasurable. Tenderness and soreness do not necessarily mean disease, it indicates that there is an imbalance that needs correcting.

- The subject may feel tired immediately after receiving a reflexology session and that is quite normal.
- Sometimes there will be tingling up the legs or a painful twinge somewhere in the body. This is nothing to worry about because it is the result of zone therapy doing its good work and indicates an improvement in circulation and energy, as well as a release of toxic material.
- Any toxic material will be carried away through the blood and lymph vessels to the excretory organs.
- It is recommended to drink plenty of water for 24 hours after a session to help with the detoxification process. Remember that water carries your positive intentions, your loving energy, your thought processes and you are 70% water!

If possible after a zone therapy session walk barefooted on the earth or grass for five minutes or more, to ground yourself and connect with something greater than yourself – Mother Earth.

The Metamorphic Technique

Metamorphic comes from the word metamorphosis. As a child (and also in adulthood) we are amazed at the life cycle of a monarch butterfly. We watch the caterpillar crawling around, observe the hanging cocoon, then wait until the day the beautiful butterfly emerges in all its glory. Nature and the life force have created what seems like a miracle and so it is with human beings. The body, if given the chance, will heal itself and reverse disease if the vital life force within is stimulated and if it is capable of doing so.

Our physical being begins with pre-natal experiences; even at this stage there may be disturbances or blockages. As we grow and move into life and various experiences as individuals we may need help in becoming who we were meant to be and to realise our full potential. This is where the metamorphic technique can help realise potential through a metamorphosis. This is a very simple method that can have far reaching effects.

Working with the metamorphic technique the practitioner does nothing to the subject but stands aside and acts as a catalyst to allow something to happen from within the subject's body. The subject's own life force moves from where it is, to where it can be - a metamorphosis occurs as old patterns and blockages move aside to allow fresh energy to begin something new from within. (*This is not zone therapy nor is it reflexology*).

During the 1960's a naturopath called Robert St. John,[60] began his work with reflexology then developed another healing art that he called the metamorphic technique. This technique worked along the spinal reflex of the foot and other parts of the body in quite a different manner to that of a reflexologist. He differentiated the techniques by saying that reflexology works by making changes within the physical body, while the metamorphic technique works on a time level and an awareness of pre-natal patterns that allow the subject's life force to bring about changes particularly on the mental, emotional, and behavioral level.

It is particularly good for children who are not developing to their full potential or people who have blocks in their subconscious which goes back to the pre-natal period of time. There is no need to go searching for reasons or to diagnose - just do the work and the body will take care of itself with whatever stimulation it receives. The subject will be stimulated at a subconscious level to make changes within their own body with their own energy. Metamorphosis trusts the innate intelligence of the subject to let go of unconscious tension and clear the way for individual potential to unfold. As the stress and tension eases the subject will naturally begin to feel a connection to the greater source of life and a different attitude to life and living will surface.

"Metamorphosis is a philosophy: it is a way of understanding the nature, the structure and the function of life in all things on this planet; but, particularly, in the human. Our origin, the reason for this origin and the way in which the original pattern changed are all points of interest and this information gives us a knowledge of what is causing the events of the present time." Robert St John [61]

Applying metamorphic technique to the feet:

Although the metamorphic technique can be applied to the head, hands, or feet, here we will focus on the feet only.

While applying metamorphic technique the facilitator must detach from any form of diagnosis or intention. This is one reason why anyone with absolutely no knowledge of anatomy, physiology, or disease, can work so effectively with this technique.

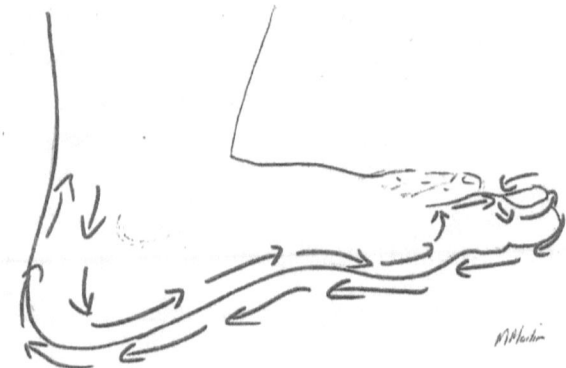

Figure 4: Illustrating Foot Zone for the Metamorphic Technique

- Always start on the right foot.
- Working on the foot the facilitator uses very gentle and soothing strokes.
- Hold the foot in one hand and use the other hand as the facilitating hand.
- When working on the foot glide the thumb or the whole hand from the heel, up the inner side of the foot to the large toe.
- Work around the large toe with finger and thumb then glide back to the heel.
- Allow the fingers and hand to go wherever they want to go.
- It's all about *glide and slide* as you apply this technique to loosen the time structure.
- If the fingers and hand feel heavy while working, remove the working hand from the foot and give it a good shake. This has the effect of releasing and throwing off stale energy from the hand.
- Continue the glide and slide for up to 30 minutes.
- Now, follow the same pattern with the left foot for 30 minutes.
- Allow the subject time to process whatever changes are occurring within their body for about a week before giving another session.

- Let the life force of the subject awaken to revitalize and regenerate from within and allow the subject the opportunity to transform into a beautiful human being.
- Simplicity and detachment are keys for metamorphosis.

CHAPTER THIRTEEN

Growing Nutritious Food

Within the first two chapters of the book of *Genesis* we read: "In the beginning God created the heavens and the earth…mankind was created from the dust of the ground and God breathed into his nostrils the breath of life: and man became a living being… and every plant yielding seed and every tree with seed in its fruit was for food… and man was put in the garden to till it and keep it."[62]

A point of interest from the creation story is about the close relationship of humans to dust and the earth. The human body is created from minerals that are all earth minerals. Among the *Dead Sea Scrolls*[63] discovered in Qumram caves during the 1940's were translations of the *Essene Gospels of Peace.* These writings shed light on the above scripture that says from dust we are created. Humans truly are made from the elements of the earth (Earth Mother) and are sustained by these elements until the mortal body is no more and it returns to the earth as (mineral) dust.

"Then shall the Son of Man seek peace with the kingdom of his Earthly Mother, for none can live long, neither be happy, but he who honors his Earthly Mother and does her laws. For your breath is her breath; your blood her blood; your bone her bone; your flesh her flesh; your bowels her bowels; your eyes and your ears are her eyes and her ears. I tell you truly, you are one with the Earthly Mother; she is in you, and you in her. Of her you were born, in her do you live, and to her shall you return again. It is the blood of our Earthly Mother which falls from the clouds and flows in the rivers; it is the breath of our Earthly Mother which whispers in the leaves of the forest and blows with a mighty wind from the mountains; sweet and firm is the flesh of our Earthly Mother in the fruits of the trees; strong and unflinching are the bones of our Earthly Mother in the giant rocks and stones which stand as sentinels of the lost times; truly, we are one with our Earthly Mother, and he who clings to the laws of his Mother, to him shall his Mother cling also."[64]

One of the most important characteristics of mankind is the mineral composition of the body. All minerals from which humans are composed come from the earth and it is indeed mankind's responsibility to look after the earth.[28] Produce from the earth is intended to provide nourishment for the human body therefore food should be grown in soil with all minerals in a balanced form. When soil is in a balanced state it will grow nutritious food, that when harvested and eaten will help keep people well.

Unfortunately, over the years humans have damaged the soil and the whole earth is affected. In many countries the cry from individuals and concerned groups is to reverse the damage done now before it is too late. We may have seen so called progress over time with the growth and development of the industrial age and modern technology with all sorts of pesticides and chemicals to enhance and produce food. However, much knowledge about the earth, and working with the earth and environment, has been lost. In many countries people are starving from lack of food and in other countries people eat far too much food. In some places food can no longer be grown from seeds and pressure is on to save seeds before it is too late.

Four big seed companies: Monsanto(Bayer), DuPont/Pioneer, Syngenta and Dow Agro Sciences appear to be a danger to humanity as they continue to interfere with seeds in their efforts to control the natural ability of seeds to reproduce. By controlling seeds, they also control farmers and world food supplies. Farmers can no longer grow from their own seeds but are forced to purchase new seeds every year with a continually rising cost. Obtaining food for the starving populations in the world is a real problem, yet if everyone worked at growing food and saving seeds, and it was shared, there would be enough for everyone.

Conversely, in countries where there is plenty of food, sickness and disease is rife, often from overeating, eating too many different foods, eating food out of season, eating processed foods, eating foods with a high sugar content, eating foods with chemicals added as a preservative, or eating foods sprayed with poisonous pesticides.

In New Zealand (and other countries too) there is a movement to try and save the planet from self-destruction by an awareness about what is happening to planet Earth, growing more trees, and cleaning up waterways. There is a growing awareness to care for Mother Earth, a mindfulness of the need to nourish the earth, and to avoid poisoning the soil with chemicals and pesticides. ***We need good healthy soil, in order for the earth to produce nutritious food.*** This growing consciousness of like-minded people provides confidence that we can work with the laws of nature, and the environment to grow healthy life sustaining foods to support life and to keep us well. In turn we save the planet.

The first and most basic step in repairing damage to our own little plot of earth is to feed it good compost in the form of humus. As compost materials begin to break down worms and other earth sustaining insects and bacteria multiply to form a rich nutritious soil. By encouraging worms to work through organic waste and compost they produce an extremely rich soil and worm juice that becomes food for plants. Plants surrounded by worms and humus are happy, they grow well, and contain a balance of minerals. Good soil is needed for survival by both plants (for good seeds) and humans (for good food).

Compost

There are many easy ways to create compost that won't cost anything at all. Any kind of compost will attract worms but add a handful of tiger worms to composting material to speed up the process. As worms start doing their work they soon multiply as they convert waste organic materials into rich nourishing soil.

Easy Compost:

- Dig a trench where you will be growing your vegetables - about 2 hands wide and 3 hands deep.
- Along the bottom of the trench throw all kitchen and garden waste, i.e. vegetable scraps, wasted fruit, scraps left over from meals, newspapers, grass clippings, and leaves.

- Add animal manure if available – pig, horse, cow, sheep or goat manure.
- Cover with a layer of soil.
- Continue to add more scraps and waste.
- Add sufficient water to keep everything moist.
- Other additions to the trench can be ground blood and bone, lime, burnt twigs and bones (charcoal), ground clay pottery or fine clay, seaweed and seawater.
- Continue to cover with a layer of soil until the trench is full.
- You may choose to plant immediately after starting your trench or you may keep adding layers of food waste, manure, newspaper etc. and leave for a few weeks.
- Ensure the trench is kept moist with water but not too wet.
- The friends of Mother Earth i.e., bacteria, insects, and worms will work breaking down the waste material and within six months you will have a nutritious composted soil where your vegetable plants will thrive.

Other methods to make compost are:

Wooden boxes

It is a good idea to have two boxes.

- Any size will do and a one square metre box is a good size for a start.
- Leave the boxes open to Mother Earth at the bottom, this allows worms and microbes to work their way up through the debris.
- Fill the first box with waste material.
- Ensure it is well watered.
- Cover with black polythene plastic held down with bricks or a wooden cover.
- Leave this box to process.
- Over the next six months the waste will be turned into compost.
- During this time water when necessary to ensure that everything is kept moist yet not too wet.

- Add grass clippings, weeds, twigs from trimmed trees, garden and kitchen waste, as well as animal manure, in fact anything that will rot and break down.
- A hinged lid is handy because this will make it easier to check the moisture level and the quality of the compost.

When the first box is full and while it is composting you can start the other box.

Drums

- Any kind of drum will do provided it hasn't contained any poisonous substance that may have left a residue in the drum.
- Cut the bottom out of the drum and make a few holes in the sides. This will allow excess water to drain out and air to flow in.
- An old bucket can be used to make compost - cut the bottom out, cut small holes in the side, and use the bucket bottom as a covering lid.

Specially designed compost makers.

- These can be purchased of various shapes and sizes.
- One on the market is called a 'worm farm' composter. This is made up of several black plastic trays, which fit upon one another.
- As one tray is filled with waste another tray is placed on top.
- Usually a starter of tiger worms is placed in the bottom tray. Tiger worms multiply very quickly and work through waste material fast.
- A tap in the bottom tray is used to drain off worm juice. The worm juice, although extremely strong, is very nutritious food for plants and needs to be diluted 1- 10 parts with water.
- As the worms finish their work in each tray they move up to the next tray. At this stage the rich composted earth from the worm castings can be removed and put directly into the garden. In this manner trays are re-used and there is always a constant supply of extremely rich, nutritious, processed, worm material to nourish the soil.

Composting toilets.

- Once upon a time, composting toilets were the norm. Nowadays, in towns and cities this is practically impossible as septic tanks and flush toilets have taken over.
- The simplest of all composting toilets is a bucket with a seat and cover over it. Two small buckets can be used to separate urine from faeces.
- The urine can be used immediately to feed plants and in particular citrus trees.
- Faeces need to be either dug into the ground, left to dry, or mixed with other compostable materials. This material must be left for six months to naturally cook and decompose.
- Larger buckets or containers can be used for toilets. Before starting with this method determine the size of bucket you can carry comfortably when full.
- Once again, leave all waste to mature for six months or more before spreading on the garden.
- Another toilet, called the 'long drop' can be as simple as a bench seat over a large hole in the ground. Beside the toilet should be a bucket of soil, sawdust, ground up tree bark, or old leaves so each person that uses the toilet can sprinkle a coating of material over the waste.
- When the hole is almost full of waste material, it is completely covered with soil and the bench is removed to another position.
- Six months or more later the mature compost is taken to the site where it will be used.
- In the meantime, another toilet can be functioning to keep the supply going. Two toilets can be built alongside each other so that when one is closed off, the other is in use.

Designer composting toilets

More sophisticated composting toilets can be purchased and there is a large selection available from retail outlets. With all composting toilets a bucket of soil, sawdust, ground up tree bark, or old leaves, needs to be kept beside the toilet for the users to cover their faeces after each use.

Other useful additions to composting materials (or dug directly into the garden are:

- Animal waste (cow, horse, sheep, or pig poo) - excellent to attract friendly bacteria and worms into the garden. Animal waste is often easier to gather up when dry. Add water to break it down into a liquid fertilizer then feed it to the plants.
- Chicken waste is rather strong but good nutrition for the soil it also needs to be broken down before use.
- Seaweed is excellent for the garden and can be soaked in water, cut up into small pieces and added to compost.
- Shells - ground up seashells can be added to compost too. A fossil shell product called 'Diatomaceous Earth' can be purchased and added to compost as well.
- Any green waste such as lawn cuttings, tree trimmings, leaves, and weeds, can be placed in black plastic bags and left in the sunshine to cook and break down before adding them to compost.
- Waste from vacuum cleaning can be added to compost. The dust and dust mites will all add value to compost.
- Old newspapers and cardboard are a valuable resource that can be added to compost too.
- You don't need to waste anything organic at all! If it will rot away, has not been sprayed or has poisons associated with it, then recycle back into the soil.

Starting a vegetable garden

If you seek to have fresh, nutritious, vegetables every day then you need to start a vegetable garden. It does not matter where you live, with a little effort and planning you can enjoy fresh nutritious vegetables from your own garden.

Let's start by discussing the city dweller or someone who has limited space in their backyard. In fact, you may have no earth around you to grow produce at all. You may live several stories up in a city building and only have a balcony. So first you will need to think about what vegetables (or herbs) to grow and where you will grow them, then make a plan. Suggestions for growing vegetables in if there is no spare ground are large used plastic milk containers, pottery containers, wooden boxes, or polystyrene trays. Any of these containers can sit on concrete or on a wooden deck.

One of my gardens was made from old wooden pallets which are often available free to take away from many retail outlets. This little garden was less than one meter wide and about 2 meters long. The base was loose stone on an old car parking area. I made the boxes quite quickly with no bottom, added compost, and planted my vegetables and herbs. I had an instant garden and continued to improve the soil by adding more compost regularly to replace nutrients the plants had taken up. Best of all there were fresh vegetables to eat every day.

When we have our own garden, we know that we are eating vegetables grown in nutritious organic soil and the vegetables are not sprayed or exposed to chemicals of any kind. If you have a large plot of land you will be able to grow more vegetables and many different kinds of vegetables. Write down where you intend planting different kinds of vegetables and how big the planting area will be as well as how crops might be rotated to get the best from them. Some plants like growing together and these are called companion plants. Decide what you prefer to eat and whether something is worth growing. With a larger plot of land, you might consider planting fruit, olive, and nut trees.

Sometimes you need to wait a few years for fruit trees to produce but it is well worth considering. Feijoa trees grow quickly and do well in most places and produce fruit within a very short time – often after 2 years. Some fruit trees require at least two trees from the same family for pollination in order for trees to produce fruit. A lemon tree is always a useful tree to grow. Comfrey and parsley are good companion herbs to grow around fruit trees but don't plant them too close to the trunk, plant one meter away from the trunk. Always have some herbs growing, they take up very little space and can be used in cooking and for medicinal purposes. Grow calendular and garlic in the vegetable garden to protect vegetables from pests.

Protect your garden

If there are animals or birds around that are likely to eat your vegetables, then it is best to fence off your garden plot and protect seeds and seedlings with bird proof netting. Trust me I know from experience! Goats, sheep, cows, and rabbits love vegetables and will chew through your garden in no time at all! Dogs and cats are best kept out of the vegetable garden. Also, hens and other feathered friends like to peck away at fresh vegetable greens and can destroy them all quite quickly and leave deposits everywhere. Either control them or let them free range around fruit trees where they do good work finding insects that may be pests. I like to grow extra vegetables, so the birds don't go hungry. Birds are good to have in the garden as they are part of the natural balance of creatures who live there and they help control garden pests.

Bees

Bees are a bonus in the garden. If you have the space it is a great idea to consider a beehive. Honey bees will pollinate your fruit and vegetables and supply you with honey. Bee hives need some attention and looking after, but you will be well rewarded as they are such a delight to watch buzzing around in their busy way collecting pollen. I love to grow lavender and other flowering plants to keep bees happy. Honey can be harvested but you do need to leave the bees enough honey to feed them over the winter months.

Bumblebees are also an option to keep in a large garden. They take less looking after than honey bees and will pollinate your fruit and vegetable flowers well too. However, they will not supply you with honey. Bumble bees and honey bees work well together doing their job pollinating flowers. Never fear being stung by a bee unless you have a severe bee sting allergy. Generally if you move gently around and talk to them they will stay out of your way. Always allow at least one dock plant to grow in your garden. Juice from a dock leaf applied to any sting will relieve the sting and the itch that follows.

What to Grow

What you grow may depend upon climate factors. However, with care you can grow anything, anywhere. A community called Findhorn in the far north of Scotland began their gardens with poor soil, a cold climate, and negative words from people saying they couldn't grow anything in that particular area. The community persevered and their gardens flourished.

Now people from all around the world visit the Findhorn community to see their prolific gardens.

Sometimes you will learn from experience what can be grown best in your area. Planning a garden is important if you want to have different vegetables available throughout the year. Some vegetables like potatoes, pumpkins, squash, garlic, and onions can be grown, harvested, and stored year around. Carrots can be left in the ground or buried in a pit, used as necessary, and they will last several months. If you live alone then you will not need to grow a lot, any excess you can always give away. One of the joys of a gardener is to give away flowers or produce.

My list of 10+ nutritious vegetables that are easy to grow are:

- Bok Choi
- Broccoli
- Green Beans
- Cabbage
- Pumpkin
- Spring Onions
- Garlic
- Carrots
- Potatoes and/or Kumara
- Beetroot
- Salad vegetables, in season grow cucumbers, lettuce, and tomatoes for salads.

Care, compost, and *water* are essential for vegetables if you want the best from them.

Herbs

Always have a small patch for an herb garden. Seven common herbs easy to grow and useful for culinary and medicinal purposes are:

- Parsley
- Thyme
- Sage
- Mint (various kinds available)

- Chives
- Rosemary
- Lavendar

Pests and Insects

Pests and insects will be attracted to unhealthy plants. Sometimes, insect pests will stay until your soil becomes balanced and healthy. Don't succumb to the temptation to spray poisonous insecticides on your vegetables. There are several natural sprays you can use to deter insects and the following are a few cheap options:

- Crush garlic, add water, and spray this mixture over growing vegetables.
- Mix natural soap with water and spray over vegetables.
- Make a homeopathic spray from any pests eating the plants such as slugs, bugs, and snails. Crush, dilute 1- 10 parts water, shake well. Take one part of that mixture and add 10 parts water, shake well. Repeat once more, strain and spray.
- Often crushing a troublesome bug and dropping it to the ground is enough to deter others of its kind from invading your garden.
- Put a plate of beer in the garden – slugs and snails will drink, get drunk, and drown in the beer!
- Gather up snail shells, roast in an old tin, crush into a fine powder and sprinkle around plants - snails will disappear.
- Dried and crushed eggshells will deter slugs and snails - they don't like crawling over the sharp egg shells!
- Used coffee grounds and diatomaceous earth will deter pests.
- Salt water – 100mls to one liter of plain water and spray over plants and insects.
- A plate of Apple Cider Vinegar will attract white butterflies (that lay eggs on cabbages), they will drink and drown in it.
- Pea straw is harsh on the bodies of slugs and snails so can be a deterrent. It will act as a mulch to retain moisture and finally decompose into the soil.

Soil

With any home garden start with your soil. If you really want to find out what elements are missing from your soil then have it analysed for deficiencies, then start the process of balancing it with minerals and trace elements. This is often a slow process and may take a few years of constant vigilance. Add only natural ingredients to your garden, such as animal manure, blood & bone, seaweed, compost, kitchen scraps, worm castings and worm juice. Encourage worms to work in your garden.

Ensure you have adequate water during all seasons.

Avoid using chemical sprays, inorganic fertilisers and poisonous pest eradication.

Consider the needs of your plants, some need sunshine, some need shade, some need shelter, rotate your garden on a yearly basis and plant nitrogen fixing plants (lupin) to enrich the soil. Strengthen your soil, strengthen your plants, eat your nutritious food and save your strong healthy seeds!

Tend your plants and trees well, love them, talk to them, breathe with them, and they will reward you with a bountiful crop.

CHAPTER FOURTEEN

Connecting to Earth, Spirit and Sound

Earth Energy

The earth is full of various energies. Energy is vibration, sound, and colour. In some parts of the world primitive people and scientists know that in particular places there are stronger or different kinds of unexplainable energy. Maps of 'Ley lines' are where energy occurs at different and more powerful rates than other places. For example, the red earth of Sedona (USA) is very beautiful and trees found growing there have twisted trunks. It is believed that this is due to a special kind of energy found in that particular region. Since visiting Sedona I have noticed trees with twisted trunks in other places in the world.

Many cultures consider earth their Mother or Gaia (Greek) and believe that if we look after her she will look after us. In fact, many clays and soils have unexplainable healing properties. Crystals and other gem stones mined from Mother Earth are sources of energy for healing practices. Wearing jewelry with gemstones from Mother Earth can be vitalizing because different stones have different colours, vibrations, and healing properties. Maifan stones contain the vibration and energy of minerals that can be released into water. These stones are utilized in the *Esuwaai Living Water* systems to release minerals and keep the water clean and clear. [65]

Judy Jacka in her book *Healing Through Earth Energies*, [66] discusses the way various mystery schools and religions view the idea of Earth as a living being and the idea that eco-systems and kingdoms of nature on planet Earth are simply the physical body of a great conscious being (S) in whom we (s) live and move and have our being. According to many teachings, humans are considered living cells in the body of this great Spirit in both a physical and spiritual sense. This consciousness associated with planet Earth is a rational explanation for a transcendent and timeless God who is evolving towards increasing perfection of all things. Ancient cultures have seen the wisdom and bigger picture whereby all the kingdoms in nature interact and evolve, not only on planet Earth, but far beyond the stars into the cosmic ocean of the unknown. Putting it all simply - at different levels the earth is full of energy, human beings(s) are potential bundles of energy, and behind all energy is a consciousness – transcendent, timeless, and eternal, whom we call Spirit, God, Jehovah, Yahweh, or some other name (S).

The simplest way to experience earth energy and utilise it for healing ourselves is to walk barefoot on earth, grass, sand, or in sea water. We experience a different kind of energy walking along the seashore or beside a lake of water than walking the streets of a city. Also, walking in the forest we experience earth energy plus energy from plants and trees with all our senses. As we connect with Mother Earth we acquire that which sustains wellness and heals mind and body and as mentioned previously, meditating and holding a biogenic battery of wheat grass is energising. Even if all we do is to look out a window and absorb with gratitude the vibration and energy of green grass, flowers blooming, trees growing, leaves of trees changing colour with seasons, or simply observe the growth of food in a vegetable garden or orchard, we will experience wellness. In our awareness we can resonate and marvel at life in all its richness and through this connection energy is absorbed into our soul.

Scientifically, we describe places of nature as high in healthy *negative ions* and positive energy, whereas energy within concrete buildings, motor cars, and other places, are high in *positive ions* which have an opposite and detrimental effect on the human body. Unfortunately, in the modern world there are many energies mankind has created and harnessed that interfere with Mother Earth and our own human electromagnetic energy fields. These affect our health and state of wellness e.g., micro-waves, X-rays, TV's, Wi-Fi, computers, and other electro-magnetic fields (EMF's).

To remedy exposure to energy fields that are damaging human body cells we need to neutralise the harmful positive ions in our body somehow. We can do this by exposing ourselves to negative ions from our environment and through a process called *earthing* or *grounding*. Walking barefooted on an unpolluted area of earth, green grass, sand beside the sea, or in the bush, allows our environment to balance our personal energy field and to keep us well. Standing with bare feet for 5 to 10 minutes a day on grass or earth will help detoxify and harmonise the body, eliminate harmful effects of EMF's, Wi-Fi, and other pollutants in the atmosphere that affect our bodies. This exercise will increase energy, lower stress, normalize biological rhythms, and much, much more. Earthing or grounding will reverse fatigue and sustain wellness, it is readily available and free. Sitting, lying, and sleeping on the earth is just as beneficial as standing or walking. All this is helped by the 70% of water in our body.

Water is a conductor of electricity and earthing allows our body to synch with Schumann resonance (7.83Hz) which is earth's own electromagnetic frequency to which we are exposed, and with which we should resonate naturally. Keeping water in our body at an optimal level enhances this natural activity. There is a lot more that could be said about earth energies and natural laws of the universe but hopefully this will stimulate enough interest for you to begin experimenting and exploring further.

A neutralizer that can be used inside a house or office is sphagnum moss. This moss is found under trees in damp shady places and is often growing in patches on a lawn through cold wet winter months. Place the moss in vases or jars around the house, particularly close to any microwave, computer, or television where harmful radiation waves might be discharging. The moss will dry out but will still be useful to deter radiation. Renew it every year.

Carbon from charcoal or burnt untreated wood is a useful neutralizer too. Judy Jacka recommends using charcoal as a neutralizer externally. Her method is to place charcoal in a plastic bag, stamp on the bag to activate the carbon, and then gently flick the charcoal bag on head, hands, feet, and other parts of the body. Activated carbon is non-toxic and should be kept on hand to use internally for treating accidental poisoning. Activated carbon is one of the ingredients in the Esuwaai Living Water purification systems.

Connecting with Spirit "S" (God)

Every human being is born with a gift from God that provides an opportunity to be of service to their fellow humans. Everyone has the potential to bless others. What makes a blessing is the positivity or light that a person emits and who bears fruits of the Spirit (S). Paul, a convert to Christianity, wrote about the fruits of the Spirit in his letter to the Galatian people. His message was written in order to bring back to faith and practice those people who were being misled by false teachings. Paul argued that it was not necessary to obey the Law of Moses in order to be a true follower of Jesus Christ. He wrote that by faith alone people are "put right" by God and that good conduct flows naturally from the love that results from faith in God. He wrote that the fruits of the Spirit were above any man-made law.

"… the fruit of the Spirit is love, joy, peace, patience, kindness, goodness, faithfulness, gentleness, and self-control. Against such things there is no law."[67]

"Immortal Mind is God; and this mind is made manifest in all thoughts and desires that draw mankind toward purity, health, holiness, and the spiritual facts of being." Jesus the Nazarene, recognized this relationship so clearly that he said, "I and my Father are one."[68] In proportion as we oppose the belief of the material sense of sickness, sin and death, and recognize ourselves connected to (S) the Spiritual and immortal Mind of God, shall we become our true individual self (s). Then we will discover health and holiness and an understanding that there is no sickness, disease, or death (unless carried in the mortal mind). It is then possible to follow, without doubting, the command to go into the world and heal the sick. This natural phenomenon follows faith from the pure in heart, supported with fruits of the Spirit, and the ability to utilize talents in whatever way natural gifts surface, as one human helps others to realise their full potential. This is a natural phenomenon that follows knowledge and is faith driven by love.

Love

Love as mentioned earlier takes many forms, yet in reality it leads back to God 'S'; therefore it is a spiritual experience. When Jesus, the Nazarene, was asked by the Jewish Pharisees which was the most important commandment of all in the law his answer was simple:

"Love the Lord your God with all your heart, with all your soul and with all your strength and with all your mind; and love your neighbour as yourself."[69]

Our Five Physical Senses, Plus One More

Our five basic physical senses – eyes (seeing), ears (hearing), nose (smelling), mouth (tasting), hands (touching), are our means of perceiving our physical reality. One other sense, intuition, is our connection with the greater 'S' and enables us 's' to tune into the great Spirit 'S' thus providing us with that sense of knowing without understanding by listening to the still small voice within. There are many ways to connect and understand this (mostly) invisible reality.

It is through our senses that we are able to experience beauty in things, for example a flower – the color, the smell, the absolute perfection. It is as if when God 'S' wanted to express beauty a lovely flower was created and often flowers appear to have little faces. We absorb and discover through our senses the wonder around us: our natural environment, art, sounds, music, birds, insects, butterflies and animals. All this is impressed upon our soul and there it leaves an image that reflects in all we think, say, and do. That's why we need to take time out to smell the roses, absorb the beauty of green grass, the trees standing still or blowing in the wind, a babbling brook, the sun, wind, or rain upon our face and be alert to whatever presents to us daily in our environment.

We are blest if we stand still, silence the mind and absorb until it becomes part of our very soul – we might need to touch the grass, pick a flower, hug a tree, or stroke an animal to communicate with 'S' through our senses. The beauty, joy, and peace experienced will then go back into the world again as we communicate with people (also animals and plants) through a smile, a loving word, a kind thought or deed. All this is love in action.

Listening to the singing of birds in the early morning or evening, the orchestra of frogs in a pond, and other sounds of nature alert us to the purity, the beauty, the absolute joy, akin to holiness. As we absorb sound it becomes uplifting and energizing – that too will be given back to the world as our spiritual vibration is expressed through our physical body. As you practice your smile, your tone of voice, your laughter, your good deeds, you will begin to see how ripples of positive energy flow from your very presence. This will become a way of life, become spontaneous and happy!

The happiest people on earth are the healthiest. Those who laugh a lot are happy and healthy. Laughing is therapy and is infectious and makes you feel good. Laugh at yourself. Often mistakes or obstacles in life can be overcome with laughter rather than becoming angry and upset with yourself or by blaming others. Conversely, anger and negative thoughts are detrimental to the self and your health will suffer. A negative situation can be changed to positive by looking for the good in everyone you meet (even if you dislike them). Just remember, everybody has a spark of the divine in them and often an individual just needs an opportunity for it to shine through. Martin Luther King Jnr once declared: "Darkness cannot drive out darkness – only light can do that. Hatred cannot drive out fear – only love can do that".

Love, laugh, and live by making your little part of the world a happy place. Like ripples spread in an ever-widening circle caused by a stone thrown into a pond, so the effect of you - your thoughts, words, and actions, can have a rippling effect in your world around you. You may never know the full effect you have on another person's life, or how you may have changed their life for the better. Everyone has a story to tell and sharing stories can be healing. Everyone has experiences in life for a reason, whether good or bad, and there is always someone along the highway of life that you can help who is in the same situation as you may have been at some time. With empathy you can go where they are and understand their situation better than anyone else because you have come through that experience and you can reassure them that there is a way out, a way ahead, even though it may take time.

Sometimes you will be in a situation where it seems the people and events around you are causing you to spiral into a deep, dark hole and a horrible negative state. If this is happening one of the first things to do is to communicate how you feel to those around you; be truthful, they may not realise how you are feeling. People differ in their perceptions of a situation and sometimes words or actions are misinterpreted, people get offended or upset, and you will never know why unless you ask or talk about it.

Everybody experiences this sinking feeling at some stage along life's pathway. Connect with 'S' and pray until you are at peace… then you will intuitively know what to do (if anything at all) within the situation.

However, to connect with 'S' may be foreign, or seem impossible for whatever reason. This is the time to connect with another human being who is kind, caring, empathetic, as well as someone who has a strong connection to 'S'. This heart-centered and loving person will help you through the difficult times. Nobody jumps into a deep pool of water for the first time and expects to swim. We learn to swim with support before we go it alone. Life is like that, there are helpers all around if we look, and once saved from drowning as it were, we in turn can help others on life's journey. After being there, now we can understand the situation another is facing. Telling our own story or just being there in a time of need, often helps others overcome the obstacles and challenges in their life.

Another solution is to remove yourself from people or situations, this may be temporary or permanent. Maybe you need to be alone beside the sea or in the bush. Maybe you need a different environment with more positive people around you or, maybe you need to change your work situation. If none of this is possible then one of the best things to do is to play uplifting music, dance, listen to motivational tapes, or read an inspiring book. As you experience or find inspiring thoughts from songs, books, or people – write them down in a personal journal. Read your notes and inspiring messages you've written to yourself, from time to time, read them aloud - it is surprising how uplifting this can be! Sound is therapeutic!

Sound Healing

Sound is around us everywhere and all sound has meaning. The sounds of nature – rippling water in a stream, rain on the roof, wind whistling in the trees, thunder crashing overhead during a storm, the sound of insects and buzzing bees on a sunny day, mosquitos hovering around on a summer evening, the sound of birds singing, an orchestra of frogs croaking, ducks quacking, roosters crowing, lambs bleating, cows mooing, a dog barking, a cat meowing, and so the sounds of nature go on and on…

Daily sounds of human laughter, crying, talking, shouting, singing - sounds coming from the human voice; sounds with emotion in the voice - of fear, of joy, of anger, of love all these sounds have meaning to both giver and receiver.

Sounds created by humans other than their voices such as playing a musical instrument, or a combination of instruments in a band, a symphony orchestra, sounding quartz crystal or Tibetan bowls, drumming circles, or simply clapping the hands; all these sounds are able to create and sustain wellness.

Two remarkable composers, Mozart and Beethoven, produced some amazing music, with incredible sounds considered divine and beyond this world. Their music still has a tremendous effect on people today. It is astonishing when you realize that Mozart never heard the rapture of his grandest symphonies and Beethoven was hopelessly deaf, yet he created superb music without actually hearing it. That leaves us with the theory that mental melodies and strains of sweetest music supercede conscious sound. Music, according to Mary Baker Eddy is "the rhythm of head and heart" and furthermore she states in *Science and Health with a Key to the Scriptures*: "Sound is a mental impression made on mortal belief. The ear does not really hear. Divine Science reveals sound as communicating through the senses of Soul – through spiritual understanding."[70]

Jonathan & Andi Goldman[71] work extensively with sound in their healing practices and through this interrelationship of sound and self they heal the inner self. Sound is viewed by the Goldman's as an extremely important practice for health - to heal the body, mind, and spirit. They view the resonance of sound as a means to create harmony within relationships too.

People create sound in many ways, either through voice or music, this influences not only fellow humans but also the environment. By playing music and singing to plants in the garden, and animals, this creates a special environment that enables them to grow well and wellness becomes a way of life for them too!

Sound is known to have a vibrational wavelength that can be scientifically measured. It is an energy that has a powerful effect on the human body. Everything within the environment where sound reaches is affected in one way or another. Sound has the ability to rearrange molecular structure. It is a well-known phenomenon that singing a certain note at a certain vibrational level can explode a crystal wineglass.

Each person's voice is unique. By using voice intentionally upon ourselves, we can heal, balance body energy, and keep ourselves well.

This may be simply verbal affirmations, a meditation mantra, or a more purposeful tuning into the body with voice soundings of musical notes. Sound can be directed to specific body regions and organs to heal. Once skilled at using one's own voice it is possible to use the voice to diagnose imbalances within another person, or an animal, then through intuition by choosing a specific note any imbalance can be corrected. This is called "toning"

Intentional use of sound

Begin intentional use of sound with a note, any note, and scan the unwell person's fully clothed body with the same note, about one foot away from the body. Initially do a quick scan moving over the entire body. It is easier to scan when the person is lying down. Where there is an imbalance the note in your voice will change. The note may change to a wobbly note, or staccato type note, but it will change in some way.

After the initial scan, stay over the imbalanced place and sound a note, it may be the same note used to find the imbalance area or it may be another note. Stay in the same position sounding the same note until it becomes clear and smooth and resonates in a balanced manner. It may be necessary to use more than one note in the same place. Scan and sound the other side of the body in the same way. As you gain experience you will intuitively know which note to use and how long to use it for sounding into the body.

If the sound irritates the subject, stop and select another method of sound therapy. Perhaps the subject has a favorite song you can sing together or listen to enjoyable music from a record.

Healing is not always about *making* sound. Listening to sound is also important as it enables the body to absorb, revitalise, and regenerate cells. A French scientist Dr Alfred Tomatis devoted a lifetime to understanding sound through music and voice and it's relationship to the nervous system. He began with a study of the ear and its function then developed a range of sounds for healing and specifically for healing hearing problems and learning difficulties. He believed that the ear was the most important sense organ because of its connections to the brain, and the nervous system of the body. He discovered that by listening to music through earphones for several hours a day it would improve the natural plasticity of the neural circuits involved in the decoding and analysis of sounds in order to retrain the brain. This was no ordinary music. Tomatis engineered classical music in a special manner that provided therapeutic effects. His methods are actively practiced throughout the world today and the ninth Tomatis® International Convention was held in Warsaw, Poland in 2018.[72]

Sound expressed by speaking in tongues often accompanies healing of the self or another. This is a spiritual experience that occurs when one spontaneously begins speaking in another language. It commonly flows from worship and prayer in Pentecostal Churches and is believed to be the Holy Spirit (S) working through people (s).

The word Pentecostal[73] comes from *New Testament* of the *Holy Bible*, and details a close relationship between the Holy Spirit and Jesus of Nazareth during his earthly life, his ministry, and beyond. The Holy Spirit descended on Jesus like a dove at his baptism in the river Jordan and in his final farewell to his disciples at the last supper, Jesus also promised to send the Holy Spirit to them after his departure. During that time, he instructed the apostles to make disciples of all the nations, baptizing followers in the name of the Father and of the Son and of the Holy Spirit, and said, "For where two or three are gathered together in my name, there am I in the midst of them." In the book of the *Acts of the Apostles* evidence of the Holy Spirit came in a dramatic manner after the resurrection of Jesus Christ.

"When the day of Pentecost came, they were all together in one place. Suddenly the sound like the blowing of a violent wind came from heaven and filled the whole house where they were sitting. They saw what seemed to be tongues of fire that separated and came to rest on each of them. All of them were filled with the Holy Spirit and began to speak in other tongues (languages) as the Spirit enabled them."[74]

Never underestimate the therapeutic value of sounds

CHAPTER FIFTEEN

Self Help Exercises

The following are ways I've kept well over the years and these suggestions may be helpful as a guide in your journey too.

Self Help Exercises:

Try to incorporate some of the following into your daily life:

- Make time for yourself even if it is just sitting in a quiet place, or reading.
- Enjoy all the gifts of nature - earth, sun, air, water, moon, and stars.
- Find a method of relaxation which you can use every day. It may be simply adding a suitable essential oil to your bath and relaxing before going to bed.
- Clear your mind through regular meditation (start with 5 minutes each day) or practice active contemplation walking during the day – this helps train yourself to think good thoughts.
- Consider growing a Biogenic Battery.
- Sit under a tree, in a garden, or in a public park with trees and flowers. Think of nothing in particular and absorb the energy from the environment as you give your breath and loving energy to plants and trees.

- Convey positive energy to others through prayer or any technique that works for you.
- Read something positive from a spiritual perspective before rising and before going to sleep at night.
- Drink adequate fresh, clean, water. Most people need to filter tap water.
- Grow some food – even if it is just greens such as silver beet and chard and a few hardy herbs like parsley, thyme and sage.
- Eat wholesome, organic, and nourishing food whenever possible.
- Find something each day that makes you feel good. It may take practice but once you are mindful of good events they appear more and more often. This may be as simple as smelling flowers or weeding the garden, or, taking up a new interest like tennis, indoor or lawn bowls, painting, singing, music, cycling, meditation, swimming, yoga, knitting, spinning or playing cards with a group.
- Don't hesitate to join a club if you want to – often the local newspaper will have events and phone numbers and many clubs provide information about their activities on their clubroom signs. One phone call and you may have found a whole new group of friends!
- Sing out loud, sing in gratitude and praise, sing in the shower, sing and talk to your animals, plants, and trees.
- If you need to be energised – go and hug a person or a tree, or take a nice long walk observing trees, birds, and flowers.
- Enjoy fellowship with people, and animals. If you are alone and lonely go out of your way to meet people.
- Meet and speak with your neighbours. Talk to anyone who crosses your path during the day - you may be able to help them in some way through just talking to them and it will make you feel good.
- Smile and be happy.
- If feeling down, visit an art gallery, go to a musical event or drama show, or watch a good film.
- Laugh a lot, its therapeutic and infectious!
- Nurture your relationships with unconditional love.
- Say something unexpectedly nice to your children, your partner, your parents, your friends even a stranger. This generally makes

you feel amazing, which in return vibrates throughout your whole body, releasing positive healthy energy for both yourself and others.

- Life is about relationships. Whether it be people, animals, or the environment.
- Think good thoughts. Say and do good things.
- Visualize yourself as vibrant and health
- Exercise daily for at least 10 minutes – any exercise at all. Dancing to music is great as it provides you with both exercise and sound therapy too!
- Take a brisk walk for at least 30 minutes every day if possible. If you don't like walking by yourself, find someone to walk with. Find a dog who loves to walk (most dogs love to walk and they need exercise too!). Any other kind of brisk exercise is good too.
- Slow intentional exercise is also therapeutic. Often following a video helps with learning an exercise routine e.g., yoga or Qi-gong.
- If possible exercise and breathe deeply in fresh, unpolluted air.
- Walking in the sunshine or exposing your bare body to sunshine for 30 minutes each day is beneficial.
- Listen to music *you* enjoy and/or perhaps learn to play a musical instrument.
- Keep a wellness journal/diary. Write down everything you eat and anything of importance that happens to you each day - your work, and people you met. Note your feelings, emotions, and thoughts. Each week re-read your entries and comment (on an empty page) after reflection, on anything negative you might change in future.
- Take particular notice of your thoughts and what you are thinking about. *Thoughts materialize.* Try to have positive, healthy thoughts and write them down. Think, visualize, and feel what you need in life for it to materialise.
- Be grateful for what you have now.
- Be positive about your progress towards wellness and goals in life.
- Celebrate your life and the lives of others.
- Give generously of time in each phase of life to help others, love lots, give thanks, have fun, and journey well!

Climb the Steps to Wellness.

Know what to do when sick. Approach the challenge of sickness with appropriate medicines or natural remedies. Don't be scared – the health laws of God 'S' will keep you safe and allow you to rejoice in your new state of wellness and a way of life you will love!

If you want to reverse disease – have a plan. This may take time and you may need help along the way, but it is possible to reverse disease and regenerate the body. *Always consult with your doctor if you are taking pharmaceutical drugs* – you may need to be monitored or prescribed a reduced dose. Don't be afraid to ask your doctor questions about the effect and side effect of any drug.

Take the first step and climb those steps to wellness - don't look back. Once on the top leave disease and the *thought* of disease behind. Many choices and paths lead to wellness. Choose your pathway to wellness with care, common sense and enthusiasm.

Grow in spiritual strength closer to 'S' and finally you will realise that all healing is available, freely given, and all you need to do is to affirm your perfect state of being.

Believe and be thankful that your spiritual self 's', the reality that is you, can link to something greater, more powerful 'S' and positively energise your whole being so that you can say *"All is Well"*. Continue to follow your chosen path. Acknowledge and develop your God given gifts. Take your steps into wellness, in service to others, always looking and climbing towards the top of the stairs, each step closer to the end of your mortal life and the path you take - into a bright shiny future - eternity!

"Then the angel showed me the river of the water of life, as clear as crystal, flowing from the throne of God and of the Lamb down the middle of the great street of the city. On each side of the river stood the tree of life, bearing twelve crops of fruit, yielding its fruit every month. And the leaves of the tree are for the healing of the nations. No longer will there be any curse. The throne of God and of the Lamb will be in the city, and his servants will serve him. They will see his face, and his name will be on their foreheads. There will be no more night. They will not need the light of a lamp or the light of the sun, for the Lord God will give them light. And they will reign for ever and ever." [75]

BIBLIOGRAPHY

Bach, Edward, Wheeler, F.J. (1998) *The Bach Flower Remedies.* Keats Pub. Inc., New Canaan, CT, USA.

Baker Eddy, Mary (1875, 1994) *Science and Health with a Key to the Scriptures.* Christian Science Board of Directors, USA.

Baker Eddy, Mary *Miscellaneous Writings.* published by Trustees, Boston, USA.

Batmanghelidj (1999), *Your Body's Many Cries for Water.* Global Health Solutions, Vienna, United States of America.

Beringer, Almut (2000) In Search of the Sacred: A Conceptual Analysis of Spirituality in the *Journal of Experiential Education.* Winter 2000, Vol. 23, No.3, pp.157-64.

Boericke, William (1927) 9th Ed. *Materia Medica with Repertory.* Jain Publishers, New Delhi, India.

Church, Dawson (2018) *Mind to Matter.* Hay House, Inc. USA

Coca, Arthur F. (1959) *The Pulse Test for Allergy.* Max Parrish, London.

Cousens, Gabriel (2008) *Creating Peace by Being Peace: The Essene Sevenfold Path.* North Atlantic Books, Berkeley CA, United States of America.

D'Adamo, Peter J. (2002) *Eat Right for Your Type.* Penguin Putman Pub. NY., USA.

Dossey, Larry (1993), *Healing Words, The Power of Prayer and the Practice of Medicine.* Harper Collins Pub., San Francisco.

Duncan, Anthony (1992) *The Elements of Celtic Christianity.* Element Books Ltd., Dorset, Great Britain.

Emoto, Masaru (2001) *The Hidden Messages in Water.* Atria Books, Beyond Words Pub., NY

Fillmore, Charles (2011) *The 12 Powers of Man*. Creativespace Independent Pub. Platform, North Charleston, SC, USA.

Goldman, Jonathan and Andi (2005) *Tantra of Sound*. Hampton Roads Pub. Charlottesville, VA.

Hawker, Sara (Ed), (2003) *Colour Oxford Dictionary, Thesaurus, and Wordpower Guide*. Oxford University Press, Oxford, UK.

Holy Bible NIV (2007). Bible Society, Australia.

Hymns of the Saints Reorganised Church of Jesus Christ of Latter Day Saints (1981) Hymn No 18. All Things Bright and Beautiful. Herald Publishing House, Independence, Missouri, USA.'

Ingham, Eunice, D. (1984), *Stories the Feet Can Tell Thru Reflexology. Stories the Feet Have Told Thru Reflexology*. Ingham Pub.

Jacka, Judy (1996), *Healing Through Earth Energies*. Thomas C. Lothian Pty Ltd. Melbourne Vic. Australia.

Jensen, Bernard, D.C. PhD (2000) *Guide to Body Chemistry & Nutrition*. Keats Pub., Illinois 60712, USA

Jung, Carl.G.(1965) *Memories, Dreams, Reflections*, edited by Aniela Jaffé, translated by Richard and Clara Winston (Vintage, New York.

Nakagawa, Yoshiharu (2000) *Education for Awakening: An Eastern Approach to Holistic Education* Vol

Owen, Harrison (2000) *The Power of Spirit – How Organisations Transform*. Berrett-Koehler Pub. Inc., San Francisco.

Roden, Shirlie (1999) *Sound Healing:How to use the Healing Power of the Human Voice*. Piatkus Publishers Ltd., London.

Saint-Pierre, Gaston and Boater, Debbie (1982) *The Metamorphic Technique: Principles and Practice*. Element Books, Tisbury, Wiltshire, Great Britain.

Szeckely, Edmond Bordeaux (1998) *Cosmotherapy The Medicine of the Future*. Essene School of Life, Los Angeles, CA.

Szeckely, Edmond Bordeaux (1981 *The Essene Gospel of Peace, Book Four*. International Biogenic Society. USA.

Sherwood, Martha (1978) *Collecting Roots & Herbs for Fun & Profit*. Contemporary Books Inc.

Teasdale, Wayne (2001) *The Mystic Heart*. New World Library, Novato, CA.

The Church of the Province of New Zealand (1989). *A New Zealand Prayer Book: He Karakia Mihinare o Aotearoa*. William Collins Publishers Ltd. Auckland.

Upledger, John E. (1990*) Somato Emotional Release and Beyond*. UI Publishing, Florida.

Vlamis, Gregory (1990), *Flowers to the Rescue*. Thorsons, London, UK.

Wilber, Ken (2000) *A Theory of Everything – An Integral Vision for Business, Politics, Science, and Spirituality*. Shambhala, Boston, USA.

Zohar, Danah and Dr. Marshall, Ian (2000) *Spiritual Intelligence the Ultimate Intelligence*. Bloomsbury Publishing NY., USA.

Website References

https//:en.wikipedia.org/wiki/Holy_Spirit_in Christianity

http://en.wikipwdia.org/wiki/Health. *WHO definition of Health* – 1948 Constitution.

https://www.health.govt.nz/our-work/populations/maori-health-models/maori-health-modelste-pae-mahutonga. *Maori Health Models*.

http://www.whats-your-sign.com/circle-symbol-meaning.html

http://www.fooddemocracynow.org

http://store.planet-tachyon.com/#l23r Tachyon products.

http://metamorphosis-rsj.com/shop/conditions.php

http://www.melva.com

Endnotes

1   *Holy Bible New International Version* (1973) Published by the Bible Society in Australia, NSA, Australia

2   Beringer, Almut (2000) In Search of the Sacred: A Conceptual Analysis of Spirituality, in the *Journal of Experiential Education*. Winter 2000, Vol. 23, No.3, pp.157-64.

3   Holy Bible NIV (1973) *1 John* Ch.4v13. Bible Society, Australia.

4   Holy Bible, NIV,(1973) *Acts* Ch.17v28. Bible Society, Australia

5   Teasdale, Wayne (2001*) The Mystic Heart*. New World Library, Novato, CA

6   Holy Bible NIV (1973) *Luke Ch.17 v 21* .

7   Nakagawa, Yoshiharu (2000) *Education for Awakening: An Eastern Approach to Holistic Education* Vol 2. Foundation for Educational Renewal, Brandon, Vermont, USA.

8   Zohar, Danah and Dr Marshall, Ian (2000) *Spiritual Intelligence the Ultimate Intelligence*. Bloomsbury Publishing, New York.

9   Hawker, Sara (Ed), (2003) *Colour Oxford Dictionary,Thesaurus, and Wordpower Guide*. Oxford University Press, Oxford, UK.

10 Holy Bible, NIV (1973: *Mathew Ch. 29 v39*.

11 Baker Eddy, Mary (1875, 1994:256) *Science and Health with a Key to the Scriptures*. Christian Science Board of Directors, USA.

12 Jung, Carl.G.(1965:345) *Memories, Dreams, Reflections*, edited by Aniela Jaffé, translated by Richard and Clara Winston (Vintage, New York.

13 Owen, Harrison (2000:75) *The Power of Spirit – How Organisations Transform*. Berrett-Koehler Pub. Inc., San Francisco.

14 Emoto, Masaru (2001) *The Hidden Messages in Water*. Atria Books, Beyond Words Pub., NY.

15 Dossey, Larry (1993:109) *Healing Words, The Power of Prayer and the Practice of Medicine*. Harper Collins Pub., San Francisco.

16 Upledger, John E. (1990:144*) Somato Emotional Release and Beyond*. UI Publishing, Florida.

17 Church, Dawson (2018) *Mind to Matter*. Hay House, Inc. USA

18   Holy Bible, NIV (1973)*1 Corinthians Ch. 15v44,53.*

19   Holy Bible, NIV, (1973)*1 Corinthians Ch. 3v16.*

20   Holy Bible NIV, (1973)*I Corinthians, Ch. 13v4-8.*

21   Holy Bible, NIV, (1973)*Romans Ch. .8v16.*

22   Holy Bible, NIV, (1973)*Galatians* Ch. 5v22,23.

23   Cousens, Gabriel (2008) *Creating Peace by Being Peace: The Essene Sevenfold Path.* North Atlantic Books, Berkeley CA, United States of America.

24   Zohar, Danah & Marshall, Dr Ian (2000). *SQ Connecting with our Spiritual Intelligence.* Bloomsbury Publishing, New York, USA.

25   Holy Bible, NIV.(1973) *John Ch. 21v25*

26   Holy Bible NIV, (1973)*Mark Ch. 16 v 15,17,18*

27   *Hymns of the Saints Reorganised Church of Jesus Christ of Latter Day Saints* (1981) Hymn No 18. All Things Bright and Beautiful. Herald Publishing House, Independence, Missouri, USA.

28   https://en.wikipwdia.org/wiki/Health. *WHO definition of Health* – 1948 Constitution.

29   https://www.health.govt.nz/our-work/populations/maori-health-models/maori-health-models-te-pae-mahutonga. *Maori Health Models.*

30   http://www.whats-your-sign.com/circle-symbol-meaning.html

31   Holy Bible NIV, (1973) *Mathew Ch. 6v22.*

32   The Church of the Province of New Zealand (1989, pp.428, 423). *A New Zealand Prayer Book: He Karakia Mihinare O Aotearoa.* William Collins Publishers Ltd. Auckland.

33   Wilber, Ken (2000:xi) *A Theory of Everything – An Integral Vision for Business, Politics, Science, and Spirituality.* Shambhala, Boston, USA

34   Seckely, Edmond Bordeaux (1998), *Cosmotherapy The Medicine of the Future.* Essene School of Life, Los Angeles, CA.

35   http://store.planet-tachyon.com/#l23r for Tachyon products.

36   Fillmore, Charles (2011) *The 12 Powers of Man.* Creativespace Independent Pub., Platform, North Charleston, SC, USA.

37   Duncan, Anthony (1992:16) *The Elements of Celtic Christianity.* Element Books Ltd., Dorset, Great Britain.

38   Dr F. Batmanghelidj (1999:172) *Your Body's Many Cries for Water.* Global Health Solutions, Vienna, United States of America.

39   Emoto, Masaru (2001), *The Hidden Messages in Water.* Atria Books, Beyond Words Pub.,NY.

40   OECD is the *Organisation for Economic Cooperation and Development* of which there are 34 member countries including New Zealand, founded in 1961 to stimulate economic progress and world trade..

41   Emoto, Masaru (2001:134) *The Hidden Messages in Water.* Atria Books, NY.

42 *Esuwaai Wellness & Energy Center*, 36 Queen Street, Wairoa, New Zealand 4108.

43 Enquiries regarding *Hair Analysis for a Wellness Profile* contact Melva at: melvamay75@gmail.com

44 Coca, A.F. (1959) *The Pulse Test for Allergy*. Max Parrish &Co Ltd., London

45 D'Adamo, Peter J. (2002) *Eat Right for Your Type*. Penguin Putman Pub. for further information.

46 For a GI list of foods see https://nutritionfoundation.org.nz

47 http://www.fooddemocracynow.org

48 Szekely, Edmond Bordeaux (1977:170-74) *The Essene Way Biogenic Living*. International Biogenic Society

49 Jensen, Bernard, D.C. PhD (2000:127) *Guide to Body Chemistry & Nutrition*. Keats Pub.,Illinois 60712, USA

50 Boericke, William (1927) 9th Ed. *Materia Medica with Repertory*. Jain Publishers, New Delhi, India.

51 Bach, Edward, Wheeler, F.J. (1998) *The Bach Flower Remedies*. Keats Pub. Inc., New Canaan, CT, USA.

52 http:// www.bachcentre.com

53 Sherwood, Martha (1978) *Collecting Roots & Herbs for Fun & Profit*. Contemporary Books Inc.

54 Odyssey, see: Wikipedia - https://en.wikipedia.org/wiki/Odyssey

55 Herodicus, see: https://en.wikipedia.org/wiki/Herodicus

56 Hippocrates, see: https://en.wikipedia.org/wiki/Hippocrates

57 For information about training to become a Reflexologist in NZ contact Reflexology NZ at www.reflexology.org.nz

58 A reprint of William Fitzgerald's original book *Zone Therapy*, printed in 1917 from the collections of the University of California Libraries is available today.

59 These two books were printed together in 1984 as *The Original Works of Eunice D. Ingham* and are available as one book today. Ingham Pub.

60 Saint-Pierre, Gaston and Boater, Debbie (1982:32) *The Metamorphic Technique: Principles and Practice*. Element Books, Tisbury, Wiltshire, Great Britain.

61 Further information about Robert St John's Metamorphic Technique see http://metamorphosis-rsj.com/shop/conditions.php

62 Holy Bible, NIV, (1973) *Genesis Ch.1v1,29. Ch.2 v 7,15.*

63 *Dead Sea Scrolls*, see: www.centuryone.com/25dssfacts.html

64 Szekely, Edmond Bordeaux (1981:36) *The Essene Gospel of Peace, Book Four*. International Biogenic Society. USA.

65 The Esuwaai Living Water System is available from www.melva.com

66 Jacka, Judy (1996) *Healing Through Earth Energies*. Thomas C. Lothian Pty Ltd. Melbourne, Victoria, Australia.

67 Holy Bible, NIV, *Galatians Ch.5 v 22*

68 Baker Eddy, Mary, (undated) *Miscellaneous Writings.* Q&A p.37 / Pub Published by Trustees, Boston, USA.

69 Holy Bible NIV, (1973) *Luke Ch. 10 v 27.*

70 Baker Eddy, Mary (1994:213:16-19, 26) *Science and Health with Key to the Scriptures.* Published by Trustees, Boston, USA.

71 Goldman, Jonathan and Andi (2005) *Tantra of Sound.* Hampton Roads Pub. Charlottesville, VA.

72 See www.tomatis.com

73 https//:en.wikipedia.org/wiki/Holy Spirit in Christianity

74 Holy Bible, NIV, (1973) *Acts Ch.2 v 1-4*

75 Holy Bible NIV (1973) *Revelation Ch.22v1-5.*

Index

T

thoughts 17
Thuja 85
Thyme 111
Thyme oil 127
tissue salts 48
Tissue salts 48
Traditional naturopath 2
traditional naturopathy 5
Tree of Life 16
Tumeric 111

U

unconditional love 14, 20, 26
Unconditional love 14
universal energies 26
urine 8, 34, 43, 79, 81, 162

V

Vegetable garden 163
Vital energy 5
Vitamins 62
voice 176

W

Water 20, 31, 32, 33, 34, 35, 36, 39,
40, 42, 90, 92, 124, 151, 171,
183, 187, 188
Wellness as a way of life 30
wellness diary 57
Wellness Model 23, 24, 25, 26, 28, 98
Wellness Profile 55, 189
Wheat germ oil 120

Z

Zone Therapy 146

www.ingramcontent.com/pod-product-compliance
Lightning Source LLC
Chambersburg PA
CBHW030435290526
45786CB00001B/297